JENNIFER JEFFERIES

F*CK
THE STRESS

THE BAM (BARE ARSE MINIMUM)
TO BREAK THE STRESS LOOP

by the same author

- ~~e Stress~~
- Th~~e~~ ~~...~~s to Sanity (2002)
- The Aromatherapy Insight Cards (2000)
- Calm Kids (2003)

F*CK THE STRESS: The BAM (Bare Arse Minimum) To Break The Stress Loop

First published by Present Day Wise Woman Productions 2024

Present Day Wise Woman Productions
www.jenniferjefferies.com
Copyright © Jennifer Jefferies

All rights reserved. Without limiting the rights under the laws of the Commonwealth of Australia and all relevant international Copyright statutes, no part of this publication shall be reproduced, stored or introduced into a retrieval system or stored in any form or transmitted in any form or by any means (including electronic, digital, mechanical, photocopying) without the permission of the copyright owner and the publisher of this book.

Disclaimer: This book is for general informational purposes only and does not constitute the practice of medicine, nursing, or other professional healthcare services, including the giving of medical advice. No naturopath-patient relationship is formed. The use of this information and the materials linked to this book is at the user's own risk. The content of this book is not intended to be a substitute for professional medical advice, diagnosis, or treatment. Users should not disregard or delay in obtaining medical advice for any medical condition they have, and they should seek the assistance of their healthcare professionals for any such conditions.

ISBN: 978-0-9752017-5-6

Editor: Amanda Jesnoewski, www.velovitymedia.com.au

Photography:
@captainsquidwizard, page 2
Hannah Jessup @hannahjessupphotography, pages 52, 136, 156
Jennifer Jefferies @thepresentdaywisewoman, page 62
Simone Gorman-Clark www.simonegormanclark.com, page 108
Jeremy Plaisance @jeeremyplaisance, page 153

Design: Ingrid Schroder, bevisualco.com.au @be.visual

Printing: Ingram Spark; Lightning Source

ACKNOWLEDGEMENT

This book was conceived, written, designed and produced in the Budjalung Nation which stretches from Yamba in northeastern New South Wales, west to the Great Dividing Range at Tenterfield and Warwick, and north to the Logan River near Beenleigh in southeast Queensland.

From the home of the nine kinship groups of the Yugambeh Language Region, we pay our deepest respect to the Elders past, present and emerging and to this astonishingly beautiful country.

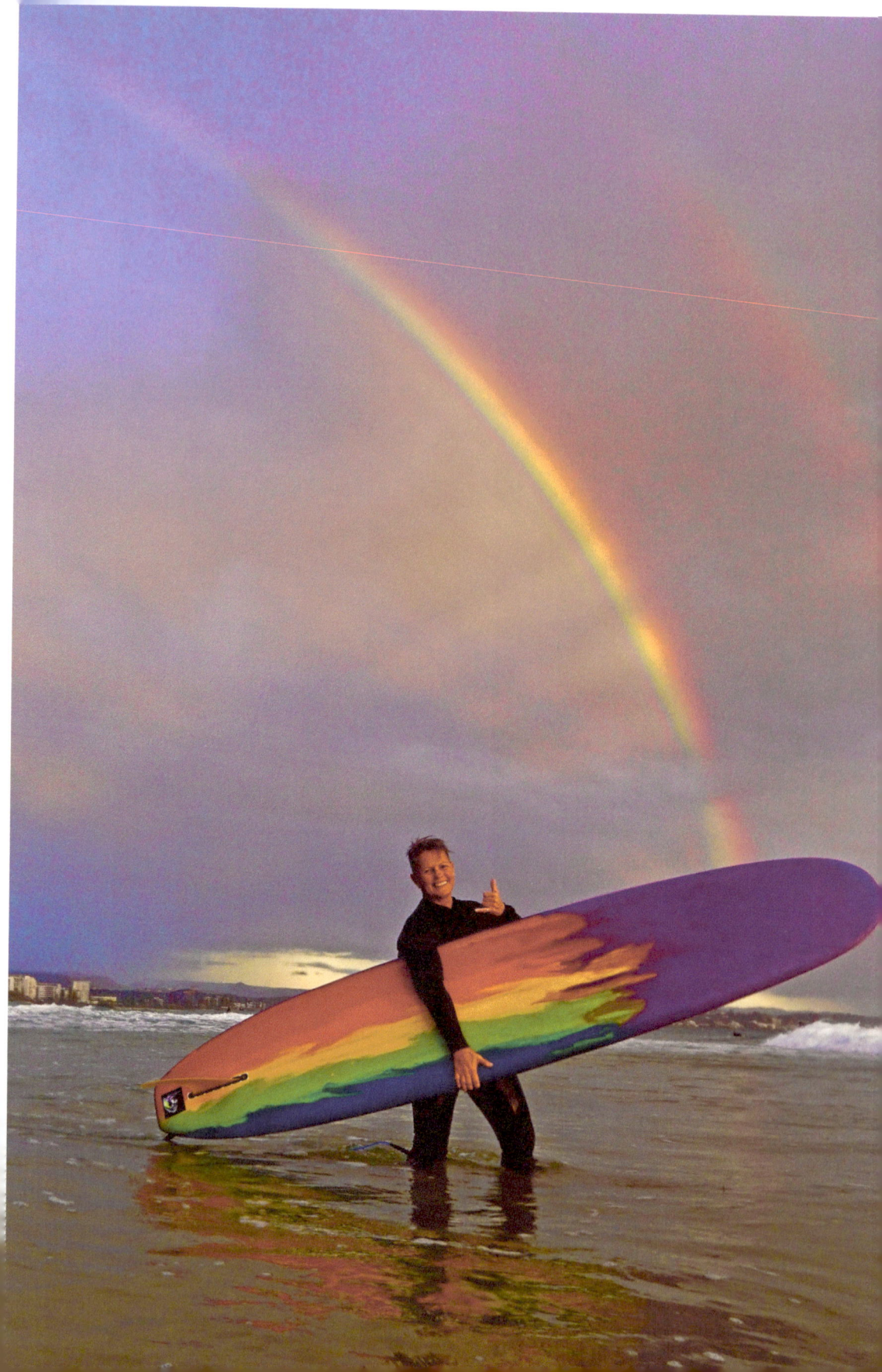

DEDICATION

To all the wise women and healers who have come before me and passed down their knowledge so that I can help others in this lifetime, I honour you, as so many of you paid for your dedication with your lives. I especially thank the courageous suffragettes, who have inspired me since I learned of your fight for our rights last century. I continue your mission of helping to build respect and advance women. I believe we can help leave this world a better place.

To my mentor and friend David TS Wood, your guidance this last decade has been life-changing for me, and I am forever thankful. My learnings from you are written in this book as they are a solid part of my mindset for navigating life now.

To my gorgeous wife, Alice Mackinnon, thank you for being the divine soul and woman you are and for always being there for me. Feeling safe and loved by you is everything to me. The thought of ageing wisely with you is the best. Bring it on.
I love you forever and always.

Contents

Introduction	**6**
Reality Check: Have you got GAS?	**11**
Mindscapes: Navigating the Modern Mental Terrain	**18**
The Loneliness Epidemic	21
Combatting Loneliness	22
Health Span VS Life Span	**25**
Health Span Versus Life Span: What's the Difference?	26
How Does This Impact Our Life Span?	27
The Triangle of Health	**29**
Our Attitudes and Beliefs	30
Our Emotional State	35
Our Physical / Situation	36
Under Pressure	**41**
Social Connection	42
Reframing the Reality	46
Seeking Support	50
The Perpetual Stress Loop	**53**
The Stress Responses	54
The Stages of the Perpetual Stress Loop	55
The BAM to Break the Stress Loop	**63**
Making the Time for Great Health	64
Self-Care	69
Good Food BAM	**71**
The Food Pyramid is a Really Square	73
Water BAM	74

Contents

Fruits and Vegetables BAM	76
Protein BAM	77
Good Carbs BAM	83
Good Fats BAM	86
Butter BAM	88
Good Sugars BAM	91
Digestive Enzymes BAM	94
Gut Microbiome BAM	96
Assimilating and Eliminating BAM	100
Intermittent Fasting BAM	101
Weight Loss and Muscle Gain BAM	106
Good Rest BAM	**109**
Adaptogens are Nature's Resilience in a Bottle	119
Good Play BAM	**121**
Mindful Movement BAM	**125**
The Window of Wellness	**129**
The 7 Steps To Sanity Condensed	**133**
Step 1. Respect Yourself	135
Step 2. Feed Your Body	140
Step 3. Move Your Body	141
Step 4. Play More	144
Step 5. Get A Life	145
Step 6. Do It Now	148
Step 7. Remember You're Human	150
Resources	**154**

Welcome to...

F*CK THE STRESS

THE BAM (BARE ARSE MINIMUM) TO BREAK THE STRESS LOOP

What if we could gain and maintain great health by doing the Bare Arse Minimum?

What's the Bare Arse Minimum (BAM)? It's what we can do to bring change to any situation. I always look for the bottom line, that bare arse minimum that a person can do to help their health. The reality is people are busy, but they still want to be healthy. This book is written for busy people who only have time for the BAM but want to break the stress loop and live in great health.

INTRODUCTION

More than two decades ago, I wrote my first book. I titled it the *7 Steps to Sanity*, as the term work-life balance was being flogged to death, yet no one had any balance. Working as a corporate speaker and trainer, I saw people lose their peace and sanity right in front of me.

If you have read the *7 Steps to Sanity*, you are already familiar with a level of the BAM approach, where you can have it all without sacrificing your health, sense of humour, or sanity along the way. That book resulted from helping thousands of patients over ten years working in my naturopathic clinic.

After ten years of working as a clinical naturopath and aromatherapist, I was frustrated seeing patients who didn't know the basics of good health. I decided to leave my clinic to bring realistic, healthy living and thinking to the masses, those who may not seek help from a naturopath but still need the information.

I see myself as the sovereign of simplicity. My goal is to demystify health and wellness and make it easy to relate to. If it's not easy to integrate into our everyday lives, we won't do it. I know because I used to write the most amazing protocols in the clinic, but they were unrealistic for today's busy world, so they wouldn't be implemented.

People don't realise that wellbeing is a skill we can learn. Professor Richard Davidson found that "Wellbeing is fundamentally no different than learning to play the cello. If one practices the skills of wellbeing, one will get better at it". As a naturopath, I agree. We learn wellbeing from our environment and everyone in it; the trouble is, sometimes, what we learn isn't conducive to wellbeing.

> **People don't realise that wellbeing is a skill we can learn**

This is how the eating habits of low-income families repeat. I remember when my grandmother passed away from bowel cancer, my mum was worried that she would die from bowel cancer as well as because it was hereditary. I told Mum that if you continue to repeat the same patterns as Nana, like eating refined and processed grains, then yes, you are setting yourself up to do that.

As adults, we can choose to change how we eat. It amazes me that we don't realise that we are allowed to eat differently from how we were raised, especially if what we eat is not working for us.

As naturopaths, we talk about our 'context'—how everything we do externally influences our internal wellbeing, and then how everything we do internally influences our external wellbeing.

When I wrote the *7 Steps to Sanity*, I shared the basics for managing stress and living from a place of prevention. Sadly, more than two decades later, and after a few significant years of extraordinary stress worldwide, stress is now even worse, and people are finding it harder to adapt or get out of the burnout hole.

This book builds on the *7 Steps to Sanity* principles and is designed to address the real epidemic of our age – stress – to guide us to a sustainable future and help us navigate an ever-changing world.

The *7 Steps to Sanity*, which include respecting yourself, feeding your body, moving your body, playing more, getting a life, doing it now, and remembering your human, seem simple. Still they are often overlooked and are even more relevant today. Sometimes, we forget to do the simple core basics that will gain and maintain good health.

69% of those surveyed are taking little or no action to deal with stress and its effects on them

In research I conducted among busy businesspeople in Sydney, I found that "69% of those surveyed are taking little or no action to deal with stress and its effects on them." This came from people saying they did not know where to start or felt it was too big for them, so they chose not to start. That's what humans do: they go into overwhelm and freeze.

INTRODUCTION

So, what do we do? That is where the BAM approach comes in. Doing BAM 80% of the time. Not 100%. I prefer a realistic and sustainable way to live. I want longevity in my health and lifestyle plan. Not some fad that comes and goes. If we do the BAM 80% of the time, 80% of our health works. We don't have to do all the big and fancy fads. What I'm presenting in this book is the BAM for food, rest, play, and movement to break the stress loop. I've also simplified and updated the 7 Steps to Sanity bringing in extra information and sharing ways that I live today. I've also included a condensed version of the *7 Steps to Sanity* at the back of this book in case you haven't read it yet. Stress won't go away and like I talk about; some pressure on us is great for our health. When the pressure is prolonged it's a different story.

Whether we like it or not, we are emotional beings living in a logical world. Today, people's emotions are all over the place because we're still coming out of one of the biggest stresses most people have ever experienced with the pandemic. It's time to get our lives back on track, get out of survival mode and start living for the future. To operate from a place of prevention so that if we're struck down with anything in the future, we'll be able to adapt, come back to the centre sooner, and not be taxed in such significant ways physically, emotionally and mentally as we are now. Stress won't go away; while some stress is good, prolonged stress is different.

> **Stress won't go away; while some stress is good, prolonged stress is different.**

So, how do you use this book? I've written it as a practical tool to complement what you're doing in life. It is the BAM. The Bare Arse Minimum. Is there more to do to live a strong, fit, healthy, active, vital life? Yes. But we won't break the stress loop if we don't get the BAM right. I find people trying to be so clever, doing all these amazing things and all they learn online nowadays, and yet we must start with the BAM. That is our foundation.

INTRODUCTION

This book gives you a practical place to start that you can build on. Open at any page and learn something that you can action, that can head you in the right direction. What I share has been tried and tested on myself and thousands of clients worldwide. More than three decades of experience have gone into this, not only from getting out of adrenal burnout but also from a place of prevention and flourishing. As I write this book, I'm 63 years old and thriving in life, being strong, fit, and healthy. That's the way it's meant to be. I know that every little thing I do and don't do today impacts my health physically, emotionally, mentally, and in the long term. Apart from being a new trendy term, biohacking is living from a place of prevention. So, what are you doing today? Let's dive into how to break and prevent the stress loop in our lives. It's time to be real about what it takes to live from a place of prevention, no matter where we are in life.

What's the BAM? The Bare Arse Minimum.

> *"Wellbeing is fundamentally no different than learning to play the cello. If one practices the skills of wellbeing, one will get better at it."*
>
> **PROFESSOR RICHARD DAVIDSON**

Reality Check

HAVE YOU GOT GAS?

In March 2020, I was in Asia on a speaking tour. The world started to lockdown with the COVID-19 pandemic, and I knew I had to return while I could. I flew back in and went into isolation.

At first, it rattled me. Suddenly, within that week, planes stopped flying internationally, events were cancelled worldwide, and my speaking income went to zero. Like so many people, I took a hit financially, mentally, and emotionally.

REALITY CHECK: HAVE YOU GOT GAS?

My life of travelling as a professional speaker for 20 years suddenly became uncertain, and I didn't know what would happen next. The world at the time sat in hope, thinking it wouldn't last longer than a few weeks, then a few months. But it went on for three years.

Now, we are seeing the fallout with a sharp rise in mental health issues. As a speaker, my speciality was talking about adrenal stress, how it impacts our lives, and how we need to adapt to it—a message that is needed now more than ever. When we can't adapt to our stress, our body fights on until it can't fight anymore.

The best example of this is the General Adaptation Syndrome, conceptualised by endocrinologist Hans Selye in 1946. It vividly describes the three stages our body goes through when exposed to stress. When I first learned this, it helped me understand and visualise what happens in the body at a physiological level.

The 3-Stages of General Adaptation Syndrome (GAS)

Stage 1 - Alarm

The first stage is the alarm reaction stage. Our body, sensing trouble, sets off an alarm. Imagine this: stress comes along, whether it's a tough day at work, an argument with a loved one, or just feeling overwhelmed by life in general. Our body kicks into high gear, activating its built-in stress response system. Our adrenal glands start pumping out hormones like adrenaline and cortisol, revving us for action. Our senses sharpen, our heart starts racing, our blood pressure rises, and our muscles get ready to fight or run from the stressor. It's like our body's saying, "Okay, game on! It's time to deal with this!" This alarm reaction stage is about getting us ready to tackle whatever's stressing us out so we can face it head-on and come out on top. This stage helps us handle immediate threats. If we don't listen at the alarm stage, our body moves to Stage 2.

Stage 2 - Resistance

The second stage is the resistance stage. It's where our body fights against all that stress we've been dealing with. At first, our body handles things okay, like everything is under control. However, that constant stress can wear us down over time, especially if we sleep poorly. Our immune system starts taking hits, leaving us vulnerable to getting sick. That never-ending stream of stress hormones, like cortisol, starts messing with our body's ability to fight off infections and deal with inflammation. And guess what? That puts us at risk for all sorts of health issues down the line, from high blood pressure to heart problems and gut troubles. When we're constantly running on empty, we get sick when we try to take a break. We come down with a cold or get sick on the first day of our holidays. We've been burning the candle at both ends, and we've ignored the alarm. That is when our body says, "Hey, slow down, take a breather, and give me a chance to recharge."

If we don't adapt and the stress doesn't cease, our body moves to Stage 3.

Stage 3 - Exhaustion

As the name suggests, this is the stage the body says, "Enough is enough!" Our reserves are empty from dealing with stress day in and day out. Everything starts to go haywire. Our body's usual ways of keeping things balanced begin to fall apart. The constant stress hormones flooding our system, like cortisol and adrenaline, finally catch up with us. We feel drained and worn out, like we've hit a brick wall, and our body's defences are down. We might feel like we're walking through mud, with chronic fatigue, feeling low and anxious, and our immune system takes a hit. This isn't just in our head. I've seen it repeatedly in my practice as a naturopath. Adrenal burnout is real. Our body reaches the point where it says, "I'm done," and we must listen. It's a wake-up call to slow down and care for ourselves, as things can't get much worse.

WHERE IS THIS ALL HEADING?

The goal isn't to achieve a utopian state of no stress. After all, comfort can kill us, too.

It's an absurdity of modern life that while stress can be detrimental to our health, so too can a lack of it. In our pursuit of comfort, we often overlook the importance of stress as a natural part of growth and resilience. Without some degree of physical, mental, or emotional stress, our bodies and minds can stagnate, leading to a drop in overall health. Stressors challenge us to adapt and evolve, encouraging physiological responses that strengthen our immune systems and enhance cognitive function. Finding our balance is key. Too much stress can overwhelm and harm us, while too little can lead to complacency and weakened resilience.

So, eating a raw, vegan, paleo, keto, wholefoods diet and drinking filtered glacial waters while sitting contemplating our navel to better meditate as we overlook the ocean from our Bali villa is not the answer. Anyone can stay calm in the temple. It's about learning practical, easy-to-implement strategies to adapt to stress so we can bring peace into everyday life.

> *Too much stress can overwhelm and harm us, while too little can lead to complacency and weakened resilience.*

The thing to get about stress is that we have a window of tolerance. The "window of tolerance" is the emotional and physiological range where people can handle stress and daily life without feeling overwhelmed. It's a concept in psychology and trauma therapy that defines the optimal zone for managing challenges and emotions, balancing stress and relaxation effectively. A simple way to understand this is how, if we get a good night's sleep, we respond to stressful situations better than when we have had a bad night's sleep. Stress, worry, overwork, limited sleep, junk foods and drinks, exposure to toxins, and more can reduce our window of tolerance. This window of tolerance can impact our alkaline corridor.

> **Stress, worry, overwork, limited sleep, junk foods and drinks, exposure to toxins, and more can reduce our window of tolerance.**

What is the alkaline corridor? As naturopaths, we say there is an alkaline corridor. This theory represents a balanced state of health. A simple way to think about it is that the human body is naturally slightly alkaline. The alkaline corridor is crucial because it supports the body in maintaining balance, or internal stability, which is essential to wellbeing.

Life has us in and out of the alkaline corridor throughout the day. Diet, hydration, exercise, and stress can influence our pH balance and move us in and out of this alkaline corridor. Stress can play a huge role in disrupting this balance. When we experience stress, whether it's physical, emotional, or psychological, our body's response triggers the release of stress hormones like cortisol and adrenaline. These hormones can have a more acidic effect on the body, shifting the pH balance towards acidity.

What we care most about as naturopaths is our level of physical and emotional resilience and how quickly we can return to the alkaline corridor after experiencing stress. Since we're kicked in and out of it all day, the ability to come back to the centre and restore balance is critical for overall health. As you will discover, this book is about having our body in a place where it can come back to centre, the alkaline corridor, sooner rather than later.

Having burned out in my twenties, I have been mindful of my alkaline corridor for over three decades now, following a "close to nature" lifestyle. I learned that our body, while it must cope, copes. When faced with stress, our bodies instinctively respond through the mechanisms of "fight or flight." This primal response is deeply ingrained within us, originating from our ancestors' need to survive in dangerous situations. Today, though, it's not the big stresses of the past that take us down; it's the continual little stresses that compound and tax our health. It's the kids saying, "mum, mum, mum", the endless stream of emails and work demands, the relentless worries about managing ever-rising expenses, and for some, it's not getting enough likes on social media. The constant little hits compound.

That's what happens and what we're seeing right now in the Western world. In 2019-22, we had the stress of the stress and disruption of the COVID-19 pandemic. At the height of it, the world was in lockdown, there was absolute uncertainty, and people were living in survival mode. Nothing was predictable, and people tried to find ways to cope. By 2023, governments worldwide decided that we're all good now. The pandemic is largely over. We went back into work and life, but people's bodies have been unable to catch up.

That is why we are now seeing a substantial rise in health challenges and, in particular, mental health imbalances. Now that the stress is largely over, it's almost like we've gone on a holiday, and our bodies are collapsing. We need to recharge. Just because the government has decided that all is well and it's time to return to "normal" doesn't mean our bodies are on the same page. Our body needs to be able to adapt to what's going on. We were still in fight and flight. For many people, the stress during that time of uncertainty was too much for too long. When you look at the GAS model, it makes sense why this has resulted, and we can see that this could continue for years to come.

> *"It is not the most intellectual of the species that survives; it is not the strongest that survives; but the species that survives is the one that is able best to adapt and adjust to the changing environment in which it finds itself"*
>
> **CHARLES DARWIN**

Mindscapes

NAVIGATING THE MODERN MENTAL TERRAIN

HOW DID WE GET HERE?

Countless studies show the impact of the years 2020-22 had on the world's people.

Forbes reported, "Fifty-two per cent of employers report their employees are more engaged working from home. Yet, absurdly, mental health concerns and burnout have skyrocketed. Nearly six times as many employers report increased mental health issues among employees since the pandemic began—burnout being among the most common."

A study by McKinsey found that one of every three employees says their return to the workplace has negatively impacted their mental health, and they're feeling anxious and depressed. A total of 59% of Americans feel more isolated since the start of the pandemic, even though 75% are living with someone, and a third are more depressed.

Mental Health Services Australia reported that the widespread restrictions of movement, social distancing measures, physical isolation, and lockdowns that were widely implemented in March 2020 took a significant toll. The sudden loss of employment and social interaction, with added stressors of moving to remote work or schooling, and the impacts of sudden, localised lockdowns to prevent further outbreaks negatively impacted the mental health of many Australians. Reporting, "The pandemic has the potential to contribute to or exacerbate mental illness".

According to the Australian Bureau of Statistics, 'First insights from the National Study of Mental Health and Wellbeing 2020- 21', in 2020-21, 15% of Australians aged 16–85 years and 20% of Australians aged 16–34 years experienced high or very high levels of psychological distress. These numbers are only for those seeking our medical system's help. Natural therapies have also seen dramatic increases in recent years. Perhaps more concerning is that most people don't seek help when needed, so statistics will likely be much higher.

The problem of anxiety and depression was always there, and loneliness was emerging.

The problem of anxiety and depression was always there, and loneliness was emerging. However, the pandemic highlighted the existing weaknesses in the system. The restrictions, fear, and loss of hope during the COVID-19 pandemic amplified what was already stirring in the community. People were already physically and emotionally stretched. It was the perfect mental health storm.

*Fear, loneliness, isolation, inability to work, financial worries, and loss of self-esteem are some of the triggers that have seen a **25%** increase in the prevalence of anxiety and depression worldwide.*

WORLD HEALTH ORGANISATION

MINDSCAPES: NAVIGATING THE MODERN MENTAL TERRAIN

THE LONELINESS EPIDEMIC

Loneliness has emerged as a widespread social issue in recent years, affecting people across all demographics. Statistical data from various countries paints a stark picture of the state of the world. In Australia, just over 1 in 6 people reported experiencing loneliness in 2022. Among young adults aged 15–24, approximately 17% of males and 15% of females reported feelings of loneliness, marking a concerning trend since 2012. Similarly, in the United States, statistics reveal that one in three people regularly experiences loneliness, with a staggering 61% of young people admitting to chronic loneliness.

As I write this, 52 countries have either a 'Loneliness Minister' or a 'Loneliness Policy' in their government.

Loneliness transcends mere emotional distress; it poses significant health risks comparable to smoking 15 cigarettes a day, as noted by the World Health Organization (WHO) and the US Surgeon General. Its impact on physical health includes a compromised immune system and heightened inflammation, which can contribute to cardiovascular diseases and other chronic illnesses.

Mentally, loneliness is linked with higher rates of depression, anxiety, and other mood disorders. The psychological toll is compounded by social withdrawal, which feeds the problem and undermines a person's self-esteem and ability to connect with others.

> **Online tools are shown to exacerbate feelings of loneliness by building superficial connections that fail to satisfy our social needs.**

In today's digital world, despite being more connected than ever through social media and online platforms, online connections often lack the depth and authenticity of face-to-face relationships. Online tools are shown to exacerbate feelings of loneliness by building superficial connections that fail to satisfy our social needs.

COMBATING LONELINESS

As an introvert, my comfort zone is to withdraw and play by myself; I've thrived on being a lone wolf. While I never personally experienced loneliness, when the lockdowns started, I noticed it impacted my normal positive outlook and mood. Something different that happens when it's no longer by choice. I knew at that point that it was time to stop hiding from the world and start playing with others, no matter how uncomfortable I was. There were a few things I did to get back into the community.

When I was 56, I took up surfing. Travelling nine months a year as a professional speaker, I scooted around the edges of the surfing community and engaged as I wanted on my terms. I knew this was an area I wanted to be more active in, so I helped pull together a women's surfboard riders' group on the Gold Coast, where I live.

During those few years, the 'Surf Witches' grew from 11 to more than 3,000 surfers. During the initial lockdowns, when we couldn't surf or hang out at the beach, I started a weekly Zoom call where we could chat and connect over a "cuppa", beer, or wine. I started this as much for my mental health as anyone else's, but we all benefited.

> *Connection is the invisible thread that weaves together the fabric of our mental wellbeing.*
>
> — CHINESE PROVERB

Another way I connected with the community was through playing my ukulele. Instead of playing alone at home, I joined a local group of musicians who meet at Currumbin Beach on Friday mornings and play for fun and community. Now, that's always my priority if I'm not travelling.

I've also recently started volunteering with the local "Veterans Backyard". This is a community gardening project at my local RSL club, where veterans like me can go, help and connect with other veterans.

Joining clubs, volunteering, or catching up with mates can bring a great sense of belonging and can help to reduce feelings of isolation. Can it be hard to put yourself out there and take the first step? Absolutely! My secret to joining meet-ups is that when I get there, I look for someone standing on their own. I approach them and say, "Hi, I'm Jen. I don't know anyone. Can I chat with you, please?" It's an approach that has always worked well for me as I generally find another introverted or shy person feeling the same way. I now have a new friendship to build on.

> Joining clubs, volunteering, or catching up with mates can bring a great sense of belonging and can help to reduce feelings of isolation.

The loneliness "epidemic" is not going away anytime soon, with people more disconnected than ever, so we can mindfully connect, engage in community and "see" others who may be withdrawing and offer a helping hand. Of course, professional support from therapists or counsellors is also crucial for those grappling with chronic loneliness or its mental health repercussions. So, it is important to get professional help if needed.

The first subject I studied as a naturopath was the state of hopelessness and how dangerous it is to our health. We need hope. The fact that there has been so much uncertainty in the world in recent years has seen the general population's state of helplessness rise.

Very soon into this change, I said, enough. I realised that the world had changed and wasn't changing again soon. While I couldn't change what was happening around me, I could change my response. There is that concept of adapting again. Our bodies need to adapt to the stress.

> *If we adapt, we thrive, if we don't, we die.*

HEALTH SPAN VS LIFE SPAN

"Stress is when the demands exceed the personal and social resources the individual is able to mobilise to adapt to the conditions."

LAZARUS

HEALTH SPAN VERSUS LIFE SPAN: WHAT'S THE DIFFERENCE?

Life span is how many years we stay alive, while health span is how many of those years we live healthy without debilitating and chronic diseases, able to flourish, and age strong, fit, and healthy. Health span is not about living forever but being able to age well.

> **Health span is not about living forever but being able to age well.**

In the "Human telomere biology: A contributory and interactive factor in aging, disease risks, and protection by psychosocial stress-reducing interventions" study, Elizabeth Blackburn, Elissa Epel, and Jue Lin discuss how high levels of stress can significantly impact telomere length, effectively accelerating the ageing process. The most concerning finding is that "High-stress women lose nine years of telomere length." As discussed within the broader context of how chronic stress influences cellular ageing.

Another study, "Telomere shortening and mood disorders: preliminary support for a chronic stress model of accelerated aging", by Naomi Simon, Jordan Smoller, Kate McNamara, Richard Maser, Alyson Zalta, Mark Pollack, Andrew Nierenberg, Maurizio Fava, and Kwok-Kin Wong, explored the relationship between chronic depression and telomere length. This study concluded that

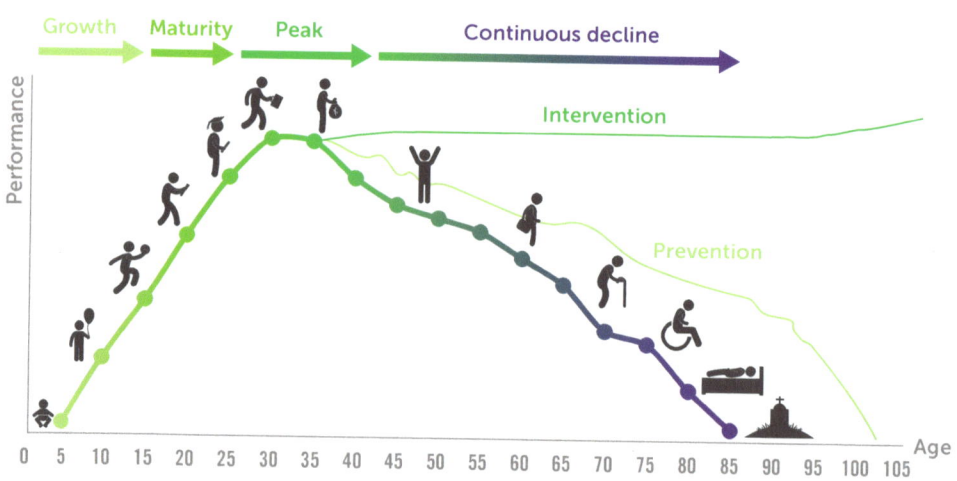

"chronic depression can lead to a significant reduction in telomere length, effectively ageing cells by approximately a decade".

So, what is a telomere? Think of a telomere as the protective little end of a shoelace. Think of the shoelace as a chromosome, where our DNA lives inside. So, we've got the shoelace with the protective little end to stop that shoelace fraying called a telomere. Why is this important?

Our telomeres are approximately 15,000 base points long when we're conceived. When born nine months later, our telomeres are about 10,000 points long. When we are about 20 years old, telomeres measure around 8,000. Now, we keep losing about 150 base pairs per year, and when we get to be less than 4,500 points long, that's when the chromosomes get unstable, and the chances of serious health problems and death increase exponentially. The things that tax our telomeres the most are physical, emotional, mental, and environmental stress. The shorter the telomere, the faster we age and the more risk we have of getting the nasty ailments in life like cancers.

HOW DOES THIS IMPACT OUR LIFE SPAN?

Being in Australia and wanting to know my prospective life span, I went to the Australian Bureau of Statistics and the UN World Population Prospects. Statistics show that Monaco is the healthiest or longest place to live in the world, at 86.5 years. Japan is second at 84.7 years, and Australia is third at 84.3 years.

As I write this, I am 63 years old. According to that statistic, the average Australian lives until about 84.3 years; I'm good. I've got a good twenty-plus years ahead of me, during which I can expect to be strong, fit, and healthy. But what they don't tell us that this is the life expectancy for people born in 2020.

So, I went and looked to see what the statistics were for someone who was born in 1961 like myself. What I found is that my average

HEALTH SPAN VS LIFE SPAN

life expectancy was 71.2 years. So here I am today at 63, and the idea of being off this planet in less than a decade does not impress me. I also live with the intention of not being average; that's why I look after my health from a place of prevention today.

Think about the statistics earlier about women who are stressed and depressed having the ability to lose one to two decades of their lives. Someone my age could be already gone. Sadly, it's happened to so many. They burned out and never got to my age. I know that everything that I do daily contributes to the longevity and quality of my life. That is why I do things daily that will help me beat those statistics, and I absolutely know that I can. That is why I'm aiming for health span, not life span.

> **Remember that health span is how long you can live strong, fit and healthy without intervention.**

Remember that health span is how long you can live strong, fit and healthy without intervention. The naturopathic philosophy is to live from a place of prevention; today, it's called 'Biohacking'. Everything we do influences us positively or negatively as we move forward. For the last three decades of my life, I've been doing interventions versus waiting to get sick and needing medical intervention. Sadly, most people wait to get sick before they look at their health. Everything in this book is what I do to increase my health span. I want to be strong, fit and healthy until I leave this planet. I will not be lingering with chronic illness for the last one to three decades of my life.

It's never too late to start. The "Window of Wellness" is always open.

THE TRIANGLE OF HEALTH

No one can avoid stress; the pressures of life affect us all. Some people may appear calm outside but they're like ducks in a pond. They glide gracefully from the surface view but paddle like mad to make it all happen below the water line — and they're causing the most harm to their bodies by internalising stress.

We can't eliminate the stressors in life, but we can learn to respond positively rather than react negatively.

Because we spend so much time at work and it's the key to our livelihoods, work can be one of the most significant and constant stressors in our lives – from the CEO's office to the production floor, we are all under pressure to perform and achieve better than our best. Being fortunate enough to have a job we love is less likely to cause us negative stress, but how many people can say that they love what they do and that it inspires and energises them? Sadly, not many. As well as doing work that doesn't fulfil us most of the time, we are also expected to leave our emotional and human selves at the door for fear of appearing weak or behaving 'unprofessionally'. All these suppressed emotions hurt our health.

Naturopathically, we view health as a state of balance between three key aspects of life. I first saw this explained by Aussie naturopath and herbalist Dorothy Hall three decades ago, and I have expanded this idea into the Triangle of Health. When the three sides are out of balance, illness will occur. When the three sides are in balance, so too is our health and our life.

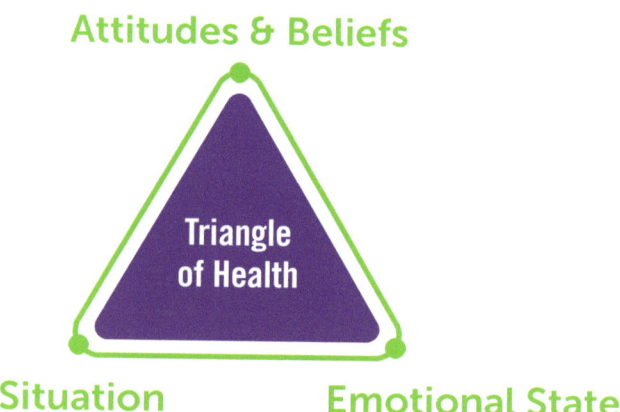

OUR ATTITUDES AND BELIEFS

Our attitudes and beliefs are subconsciously formed by observations, experiences, and other influences. We are often unaware of them, but they wait in our subconscious, ready to be used when the conditions are right. These attitudes and beliefs have a strong influence our physical and emotional health.

We've all had the experience, despite our best efforts to avoid it, where we hear ourselves say something and sound just like our mother or father did when we were kids. We vowed we'd 'never end up like that', so how did it happen? Our parents' beliefs and attitudes get hard-wired into our subconscious during our formative years. Despite our conscious desires, they are deeply ingrained and influence our own beliefs and attitudes.

Have you ever heard the saying 'whatever we resist, persists'? The more we focus on trying not to be like our parents, in this instance, the more we find ourselves becoming just like them. Similarly, the more we focus on trying not to get stressed, the more stress we will experience because that has become the focus of our attention. Our subconscious mind gets bombarded with messages about what we don't want and doesn't hear the 'try not to' part. So, the first thing to do is to recognise the pattern and understand how our subconscious mind works and affects us. Instead of focusing on trying not to be stressed, we can switch our focus to being calm and relaxed. This sends the right instructions to our subconscious mind, and we find ourselves suddenly doing what we knew we could do now that we feel calm and relaxed. The power move is to focus on what we want, not what we don't want.

> **Instead of focusing on trying not to be stressed, we can switch our focus to being calm and relaxed.**

In the same way that we find ourselves taking on behaviours we don't want by focusing on the wrong things, we can also take on adverse health by focusing on the wrong things. I remember one client who came to me convinced that she was going to get high blood pressure because her mother had it. She was an intelligent woman and business owner. I asked her a lot of questions about her lifestyle and her mother's lifestyle, and what I found was that she was repeating many of the same health habits that her mother did and was living the type of life that would lead anyone to develop high blood pressure – family history or not.

Her firm belief that she would end up with high blood pressure was leading her to the exact type of behaviours that would guarantee it. Another example of a belief manifesting adverse health outcomes that we might recognise in ourselves or someone we know is the old 'I always get a cold, at least once a year'. This is a direct instruction to our subconscious mind to make it happen.

In the book The Expectation Effect, David Robson says it best, "The power of expectation is not in what we hope for, but in what we believe is possible." The kicker is that a belief is a thought that we have over and over.

In the book Your Mind Can Heal You, Frederick Bailes writes:

> *The body itself has no power to generate illness; illness is merely the shadow thrown by the mind. A healthy mind will shadow forth a healthy body; an unhealthy mind will shadow forth an unhealthy body. Every new cell created in the body is either a negative or a positive thought in form. In the older days, it was customary to say that cells are 'built under the influence' of either negative or positive thought. In reality, the cells are the thought itself. Healthy thoughts mean healthy cells; sick thoughts mean sick cells.*

We do so many things in life operating on autopilot. We don't consciously recognise what we are doing and why or how it's impacting us, we act out behaviours based on the attitudes and beliefs we have subconsciously gathered. As we can now begin to understand, these subconscious beliefs can sabotage us from achieving the outcomes we consciously desire. So how do we correct it? Unfortunately, there's no quick fix. It's about gradual behavioural change, which begins by living consciously. The most effective method of achieving this that I have found with my clients is to have them

> **Unfortunately, there's no quick fix. It's about gradual behavioural change, which begins by living consciously.**

catch themselves off track and reward themselves for noticing. However, most people catch themselves off track, give themselves a hard time and feel guilty about their negative behaviour. But that reinforces more negative behaviour.

Think about this. We all know that eating an entire packet of chocolate biscuits in one sitting is not nutritionally balanced. Yet one evening, after a particularly challenging day at the office, we find ourselves halfway through the packet. Our first reaction is guilt, disappointment, disgust and maybe even self-loathing, but we figure the damage is done, so we might as well finish the whole packet and start on the healthy living program again tomorrow. After all, it's impossible to begin living well with half a packet of chocolate biscuits in the house! If chocolate biscuits aren't your thing, it could be a bottle of wine or a six-pack of beer.

How would the situation be different if, having found ourselves halfway through the biscuit packet, bottle, or six-pack, our reaction was positive instead of punishing? What if we acknowledged ourselves for stopping halfway through rather than finishing the lot like usual? Punishing ourselves emotionally only compounds the negative impact on our bodies. The effect of the emotional stress that comes from guilt or regret over not doing the things we know we could create more psychological pain and physical damage than whatever we ate was ever going to. Whenever we experience an overload of emotional stress, the emotions that come with it set off acidic and inflammatory reactions, releasing free radicals and a host of other negative physical reactions in our body. When we notice that we're off track, we shouldn't negatively reinforce our behaviour by punishing and guilt-tripping ourselves. Instead, we can acknowledge what we noticed, replace our negative attitude or belief with a positive and constructive one, and get back on track. I say, "Off track, back on track". No story. No problem.

> **When we notice that we're off track, we shouldn't negatively reinforce our behaviour by punishing and guilt-tripping ourselves.**

THE TRIANGLE OF HEALTH

Punishing ourselves emotionally only compounds the negative impact on our body. I say to myself, "off track, back on track".

No story. No problem.

OUR EMOTIONAL STATE

The second point of the triangle is our emotional state. In naturopathy, we take a person's emotional state seriously. Prolonged stress and negative emotions can bring a person to a state of helplessness, which increases their susceptibility to illness.

In 1975, Dr Martin Seligman, at the University of Pennsylvania, was conducting a study into escape behaviour in dogs but instead accidentally discovered the Theory of Learned Helplessness. Dr Seligman placed the dogs into a box that was divided in the middle. When the dogs jumped from one side of the box to the other, they received a small electric shock. After experiencing repeated shocks, the dogs quickly stopped trying to jump from one side to the other. The next day, the experiment was modified so there was no shock, but most dogs didn't even try to jump to the other side – they just lay down and whined. They had learned helplessness. Elephant trainers have used the theory of learned helplessness to significantly restrain these powerful creatures with nothing more than a rope or chain that a grown elephant could easily break. When the elephants are small, they are restrained with a rope or chain tied to a small tree or stake, which at that stage does restrain them. As the elephant grows it quickly becomes physically powerful enough to escape its restraint, but it has learnt that the chain or rope prevents it, so it stops trying. The chain becomes a psychological restraint rather than a physical one. The same is often true of people. We learn helplessness based on past experiences that bind us powerfully to beliefs that it's all 'too hard' or behavioural habits such as the 'poor me' syndrome, which affects our thoughts, beliefs, behaviours and health. And sooner or later, something must give.

> **We learn helplessness based on past experiences that bind us powerfully to beliefs that it's all 'too hard'**

In my former life in the corporate world, it took a serious car accident to make me stop and listen to what my body had been trying to tell me. I hadn't been paying attention for years. I thought I could do it all, and like most people, I relied on stimulants such as caffeine, food, and alcohol to give me the energy and brain space to keep going. In those days, I always had something physically wrong with me. Now I know why. I kept suppressing the negative emotions I was feeling, so my negative emotions kept showing up in my physical health. I now know that my choice of how to respond to the circumstances of my life will determine the outcome, both emotionally and physically.

> *"Expectations determine outcome, always!"*
>
> DEEPAK CHOPRA

OUR PHYSICAL / SITUATION

Have you ever wondered how it is that we end up in the same situations again and again throughout our lives? Perhaps we find ourselves in high-stress work environments, or working with people we find challenging and confronting. Maybe we repeat the same relationship patterns again and again, or we might be someone who is always 'broke' or struggling with one health issue after another. Our life's physical and situational aspects form the third point of the triangle. One perspective is that the circumstances of our lives are what they are, and we don't have influence them. Another is that subconsciously, we contribute to our situation by seeking out familiar circumstances and events that give us some emotional payoff.

In Love Your Disease, Dr John Harrison explains that people contribute to the state of their physical health to the extent that they manifest conditions that help them meet their emotional needs. The same applies in all aspects of life – perhaps we subconsciously seek out stressful work environments to fulfil a need for people to admire our ability to cope or to feel sorry for our situation. Wherever we are in our life today and whatever we are experiencing, it is of our choosing, and whether we can consciously recognise it or not, we're getting some payoff for it.

The big question is, what payoff are we getting from our current life situation and the things that stress us? That's a confronting question that we might reject by refusing to accept that we are contributing to our situation, and that's okay. We can park it in the back of our minds and return to it the next time we find ourselves at a crisis point. It's worth reflecting and noticing how we are moving forward.

> **As professional, sophisticated grown-ups, we don't want to admit to ourselves or others that we need that sort of love.**

From the time we are children, we learn that we seem to get the most love and attention when we are unwell. As professional, sophisticated grown-ups, we don't want to admit to ourselves or others that we need that sort of love and attention, and we don't know how to ask for it. But subconsciously, we know that if we are unwell, we can be looked after and cared for the way we want. My wife and I have learnt all about the sympathy and attention game, and we refuse to play it with each other. If either of us is experiencing an ailment or hurts ourselves, we quiz each other about what we were thinking at the time and why the illness or injury has manifested. From there, we can determine what purpose it serves and what we need, and were too afraid to ask for it. It has improved our health and relationship because we don't do anyone any favours by playing into their 'poor me' attention seeking. The next time you're struck down with an ailment, you can ask yourself what else in your life may have caused enough stress to manifest or exacerbate it.

What payoff are we getting from our current life situation and the things that stress us?

There is always a payoff.

AN EXAMPLE OF AN OUT-OF-BALANCE TRIANGLE OF HEALTH

When I was a child, I was always 'snotty' and on penicillin, I have vivid memories of my mother pushing little yellow tablets down my throat because I always had some respiratory infection. I can even smell the pasty aroma of those tablets, thinking about it now. I grew up believing that my sinus and hay fever came from being allergic to cats and pollens. Over the years, sure enough, I was always full of snot whenever it was wattle season or when we visited someone with a cat. Then, when I started studying natural therapies, I began to track when my bouts of hay fever and sinus would occur, and I found that they always happened when one of two things was going on in my life. The first was when something was coming up that I didn't want to do and the second was when something didn't go how I wanted it to – it literally 'got up my nose'. This was a huge realisation for me, and I began to understand how I was responsible for my health.

Relating this to the Triangle of Health, my allergy to cat hair was based on a belief that I was allergic to cats. I had that belief because when I was 12, I asked my mum for a cat and she told me I couldn't have one because I'm allergic to them. I had all the evidence to back that statement up, too, with my long history of hay fever and sinus. That was the 'beliefs' side of the triangle. If we were visiting someone I didn't want to visit, and they happened to have a cat, Mum would reinforce that belief by reminding me. The 'physical' side of the triangle was the cat hair, and my stress about visiting that person was the 'emotional' side. The bottom line is that I didn't want to visit the person with the cats. As a kid, I didn't know how to say that, so I suppressed my emotions. The stress of that manifested more snot than anyone could believe. My triangle meeting the

> **We learn helplessness based on past experiences that bind us powerfully to beliefs that it's all 'too hard'**

THE TRIANGLE OF HEALTH

three sides in a negative place gave me the symptoms and then reason to be able to sit quietly alone while the family did their visit. Did I do it consciously? No. We are emotional beings, and we all hold stress somewhere in our bodies. For me, it's my nose. For some, it's headaches, back pain, or upset stomach; we all have our physical stress default.

> **We are emotional beings, and we all hold stress somewhere in our bodies.**

The reality is that I never was allergic to cats, but I believed I was, so I experienced all the physical symptoms of someone who was allergic. Decades later, I asked my mother why she told me I was allergic to cats, and she told me it was because she didn't like cats. I took on her belief, and it was impacting my health. Today, I love cats and dogs and have my own. Occasionally, I still experience hay fever and sinus, but now, when I notice the first symptoms, I look at what else is happening around me and how I'm handling it. I can then reframe my mind about what's going on, which breaks the negative pattern, settles the symptoms and returns all points of the triangle to a positive state and balance.

> *"Every experience that we have is unique to us because at some deep level we make an interpretation of it."*
>
> **DEEPAK CHOPRA**

UNDER PRESSURE

Tennis icon Billie Jean King is famous for the quote, "Pressure is a privilege. It only comes to those who earn it."

This quote reflects her belief that pressure is not something to be feared but rather a sign of opportunity and success. I agree. Pressure is a natural part of life and achieving our goals.

It is our choice to view the pressure of stress as positive or negative in our lives.

SOCIAL CONNECTION

The Harvard Study of Adult Development, spanning a massive 73 years, has provided profound insights into the factors influencing healthy ageing. Among its most exciting findings is the importance of social connections and relationships in promoting longevity and overall wellbeing. The study reveals that people who maintain close relationships—whether with family, friends, or community—are happier and healthier as they age. These connections act as a buffer against life's stresses, helping to reduce the impact of stress hormones like cortisol and develop a sense of purpose and fulfilment.

The study shows that it is the quality, rather than the quantity, of relationships that is essential to healthy ageing. Meaningful connections characterised by trust, empathy, and support have been linked to better cognitive function, physical health, and emotional resilience in older adults. The research shows the profound impact that nurturing relationships can have on our ability to cope with life's challenges and enjoy a fulfilling and prolonged life span.

> **Meaningful connections...have been linked to better cognitive function, physical health, and emotional resilience in older adults.**

During the pandemic, isolation was a reality. Communities and families were separated for weeks, months and, for some, years. I live in a border town, and a hard border was established in hours. We all live and operate daily on both sides of the border. When this was announced, it meant a mad scramble to 'get home' to our right side of the invisible border. Hard barricades were eventually put up and many did not make it in time. The result, kids were stuck on the 'wrong side' of the border with friends and didn't see their family for months. People lost their jobs as they lived on one side and worked on the other side and were unable to cross the border to work.

During that time, three events that changed this lone wolf's way of being forever.

The first was sitting in the back of Brenda's surf van one cold winter morning. Brenda was a surfing mate who lived in Queensland and worked just across the border. She couldn't get to work, and it felt like she was lost. In the moment when she first told me, I felt helpless and knew I needed to be there for her. Like for myself and so many people, apart from the financial burden of not working, her mental health, self-esteem, and everything was rattled. I made it a priority to keep an eye out for her. I love that it brought our friendship even closer and helped me be a more present and mindful friend. The early morning 'sneaky' chats in her van are still treasured memories today. We knew that the world had changed; we were working it out together, and we realised it was so important to come together and live mindfully of the mental health of others in our community From my conversations with Brenda, I started the weekly Zoom meetings for the women I surfed with. We could jump on just chat and have a cuppa or a beer. After all, if this happy lone wolf felt the need to stay connected, then surely others also needed to.

The second, I remember when there was a 15-minute boundary that we were not allowed to cross. We could not drive further than 15 minutes from our home. I lived at the northern end of the Gold Coast and generally surfed the southern end of the coast, more than half an hour's drive away. With police checks everywhere, I decided to stay in my zone. A couple of other of our surf girls, Minxy and Mel, lived even further away. When the restriction was lifted at 4pm on a Sunday, the three of us who lived furthest away decided we needed to see each other and surf right then. Our mates had still been surfing our favourite point break in their area at Currumbin Alley, and we missed them dearly. The countdown was on, and at that minute the three of us hightailed it to "the alley". When we were back surfing, we heard screams and yahoos from three gorgeous mates, Kylie, Nana and Skye, who had come down just to love on us being able to surf again. The joy in the air was palpable. After we surfed, we hung out, ate pizza in the rain and had the best time. When that happened, I started to question what being a lone wolf was costing me in the way of connection.

> **I started to question what being a lone wolf was costing me in the way of connection.**

The third was a game-changer for me. Some of our surfing girls were on the other side of the border, and we hadn't seen them for months. I'll never forget the first "One Wave" group mental health support surf once the borders opened. When one of the girls, Kasey, arrived at the beach, it was like Christmas morning, we all ran and screamed and hugged her like no other. Emotions were high, and there were tears of joy. It was like we had been separated from family.

As a result of those three events, this lone wolf decided it was time to come in from the cold and become part of the pack. Our group, Surf Witches, has shown me what being in a community means. Being connected to them during a pandemic, the lockdown, and the isolation helped me maintain my sanity. It hasn't always been easy, as my default for my life has been to 'go my own course', but the positive impact on my mental and emotional health has been priceless. I get more comfortable as time passes, and I crave and treasure my time with these women. They are family to me.

You might be thinking, yes, Jen, the pandemic happened, but we are down the track from there. Let's move on. Some of us can and have, yet statistics show that many people have not been able to.

The Blue Zone, a show on Netflix, it was revealed that the secrets to ageing well and increasing our health span were eating wisely, having a positive outlook, making movement a habit, having a purpose in life, and connecting with others as often as possible. Yes, we are social beings, and connection keeps us alive.

> *Regardless of age, everyone in the blue zones forms genuine connections with members of their community. It's the most critical commonality between all the blue zones, and likely the most impactful secret to longevity.*
>
> "THE BLUE ZONE" NETFLIX

REFRAMING THE REALITY

Anytime that we are challenged on any level, our mind will aim to step in to help us make sense of and deal with whatever the challenge is. Depending on our past, that default will be more of a survival crisis or standing strong, knowing we can handle it.

Growing up, I had challenges and tended to expect the crisis to escalate. However, in mindfully growing myself over the past few decades, I have taught my mind to choose possibility over tragedy.

> **I have taught my mind to choose possibility over tragedy.**

When I flew back to Australia in 2020 after speaking overseas, the pandemic was unfolding. I had a choice to default to panic and doom or to possibility. For a short while, I defaulted to doom, and I felt resigned and cynical. I was watching the mainstream news and buying into the fear. The crazy thing is that I normally would never watch the news. One day, I said enough, and I stopped. I knew this was not the way I wanted to feel.

I know that nothing means anything unless I give it meaning. There is an event, which can be positive or negative, and then there is my response to it. Depending on my response and my giving it a particular meaning, I experience stress or pleasure.

So, how did I reframe and get out of that funk? What we think about, we bring about. With so much fear and uncertainty around the pandemic, it was easy to go down the rabbit hole, building those feelings of anxiety and despair.

My mentor, David TS Wood, taught me over a decade ago that Event + Story = Problem, or Event + No Story = No Problem. Technically, this is called cognitive reframing. As a naturopath, I learnt it when studying subjects like Kinesiology. When a person has an event or trauma that has locked physically into their bodies with a physical symptom, we work with the patient to help reframe the person's point of view to one of more positive.

UNDER PRESSURE

Early into 2020, I was faced with the reality of not travelling nine months of the year like I was used to and being home-based for my work. I chose to focus on the possibilities of that instead of the drama of it. Now, that took some mighty mindful work, as initially, I grieved what I was missing in terms of income and the lifestyle of being paid to travel the world. But the reality was that now I had so much more time to focus on other pursuits, like learning to surf. I went from a beginner to an intermediate surfer, which I am stoked about. My surfing was fast-tracked by my being at home more and being able to practice.

> **How did I reframe my mind? I knew I needed to stop feeding it the doom and gloom.**

How did I reframe my mind? I knew I needed to stop feeding it the doom and gloom. I switched off the news and was mindful of what I let into my thoughts through books, podcasts and people. I knew I needed some accountability. I needed to surround myself with other upbeat women who I could be there for, and they could be there for me. I love sunrise, so by going to the beach daily for a sunrise surf (yes, that's my preferred time to surf), I started to see other women who were surfing at a similar level to me. We chatted and grew into a community of over 3,000 women surfers who have formed a women's surfboard riders club, The Surf Witches Board Riders Club. Along with two of the other surfers, Hannah and Kelly, we started playing with the idea of forming a club and I became the founding president. Today, I am surrounded by this amazing, supportive community of women I would never have deeply connected with if I had continued travelling as much as I had.

So, I had a choice:

Event + Story (fear, uncertainty and making no money)
= **Massive stress and overwhelm.**
Or
Event + No story (stop what wasn't working, focus on what I love doing, and make connections with others)
= **Something incredible** that I would never have achieved if I'd kept travelling that much.

F*CK THE STRESS: THE BAM (BARE ARSE MINIMUM) TO BREAK THE STRESS LOOP

Not travelling as much also made room in my life to allow a new partner the space to come in. I had longed for a committed, loving relationship and had been struggling with dating. With the travel demands, I never realised there was no space for a partner. I used the time I gained from a lack of travel to work on myself and what I truly wanted. This all helped prepare me for my now wonderful surfer girl wife, Alice. I now had the mind and emotional space to live in a relationship mindfully.

Ironically, 2020-22 ended up being three of the best years of my life. Was my day-to-day life different? Yes. Did work and earning an income sort itself out? Absolutely it did. Did I end up being eternally thankful for it? Yes.

Was it easy to reframe it in the moment? No. However, it did help to know that I needed to adapt as the world being locked down would not resolve quickly. The bottom line is that I searched for a different perspective. I stuck to the facts, no story, no problem.

> **I searched for a different perspective. I stuck to the facts, no story, no problem.**

The facts were that I couldn't attend conferences face-to-face and speak like I had done for the previous twenty years. But I could still speak online and customise my services to the new challenges people in the workplace were finding.

The event, with no negative fear-based story attached, meant I could keep moving forward rather than being immobilised. Did I still lose most of my income? Yes. Did I have the opportunity to adapt my business to the new hybrid working landscape? Yes, and that brought me so many benefits, like so many other people now days. The pandemic went on for long enough that I, too, adapted, and I do not want to return to the amount of travelling I was doing. If this had been suggested to me at the end of 2019, I would never have believed you, and I would never have said that I wanted to roll back my travelling, as I loved it so much.

This is why I love the saying, "What we think about, we bring about".

If we think life sucks...it will.

If we think it rocks...it will.

Our thoughts help create our future. Our thoughts create our feelings, our feelings create our actions, and our actions create our results. So, if we don't want a crap result, we need to stop thinking crap thoughts. Then we won't be a crap magnet.

> **Our thoughts create our feelings, our feelings create our actions, and our actions create our results.**

We never know what will happen next. We live in less predictable times now, and we get to adapt and grow. Like in nature, nothing is stagnant.

Event + Story = Problem
Event + No Story = No Problem.

DAVID TS WOOD

UNDER PRESSURE

SEEKING SUPPORT

Asking for help is such an important lesson today. I have so much respect for those who ask for help. Why? Because I know how hard it can be to ask for help. I have been mindfully living the practice of asking for help for more than three decades. If we were drowning, we wouldn't hesitate to scream out for help. Yet, when life is on top of us, we don't. How crazy is that?

Humans are service-oriented beings, and when we ask for help, we allow others to feel of service. Studies show that giving back to others boosts our happiness, health, and sense of wellbeing. Yet we get stuck on our ego and are selfish, not allowing the other person to enjoy the good feelings when we let them help us.

> So, what stops us from asking for help? The bottom line is our ego.

So, what stops us from asking for help? The bottom line is our ego. Our ego and our false pride stop us. I learned this lesson about twenty years ago when a colleague of mine could see I was struggling with a pitch for a corporate gig. I didn't know how to pitch for that level of event and didn't want to ask for help. I thought I could work it out. But the reality was that I was wasting time and would miss out on the opportunity. I remember squirming in the most horrible feelings of not being worthy or feeling good enough. I was embarrassed and ashamed. I knew I needed to ask for help, but my ego wasn't letting me. What was remarkable was that my colleague could see what was happening and left me to squirm by not jumping in and asking if she could help Eventually, I took a deep breath and said, 'I don't know how to do this, can you help me, please?' Of course, she said yes and it changed my way of being altogether. I felt it to my

> Eventually, I took a deep breath and said, 'I don't know how to do this, can you help me, please?'

core that I could do so much more if I parked my ego and pride and asked for help.

How do I manage asking for help now days? I don't see asking for help as a weakness; I see it as a decisive move essential to my wellbeing. I see it as an act of strength. I ask from my heart, and I gratefully receive the help.

As much as I had written and taught about stress and the stress response for decades before the pandemic, asking for help is far more important than I had ever given attention to before 2020.

If you need professional help, get it, whatever your style. I'm into kinesiology as my preferred method of moving stuck emotions. Whatever your stress management strategy is; just use it, and please always remember to factor in asking for help.

> If you need professional help, get it...Whatever your stress management strategy is, use it.

My wife Alice also practices a form of body-and-energy-based support (as kinesiology is) called Evidence-Based Emotional Freedom Technique (EFT), commonly known as Clinical Tapping. It's a powerful form of real-time, real-life stress reduction and can also be used therapeutically 1-1 for things like being stuck, pain, anxiety, depression, PTSD, emotional eating, and food cravings. It's also a great tool for setting goals and removing doubts and mental obstacles to your goals.

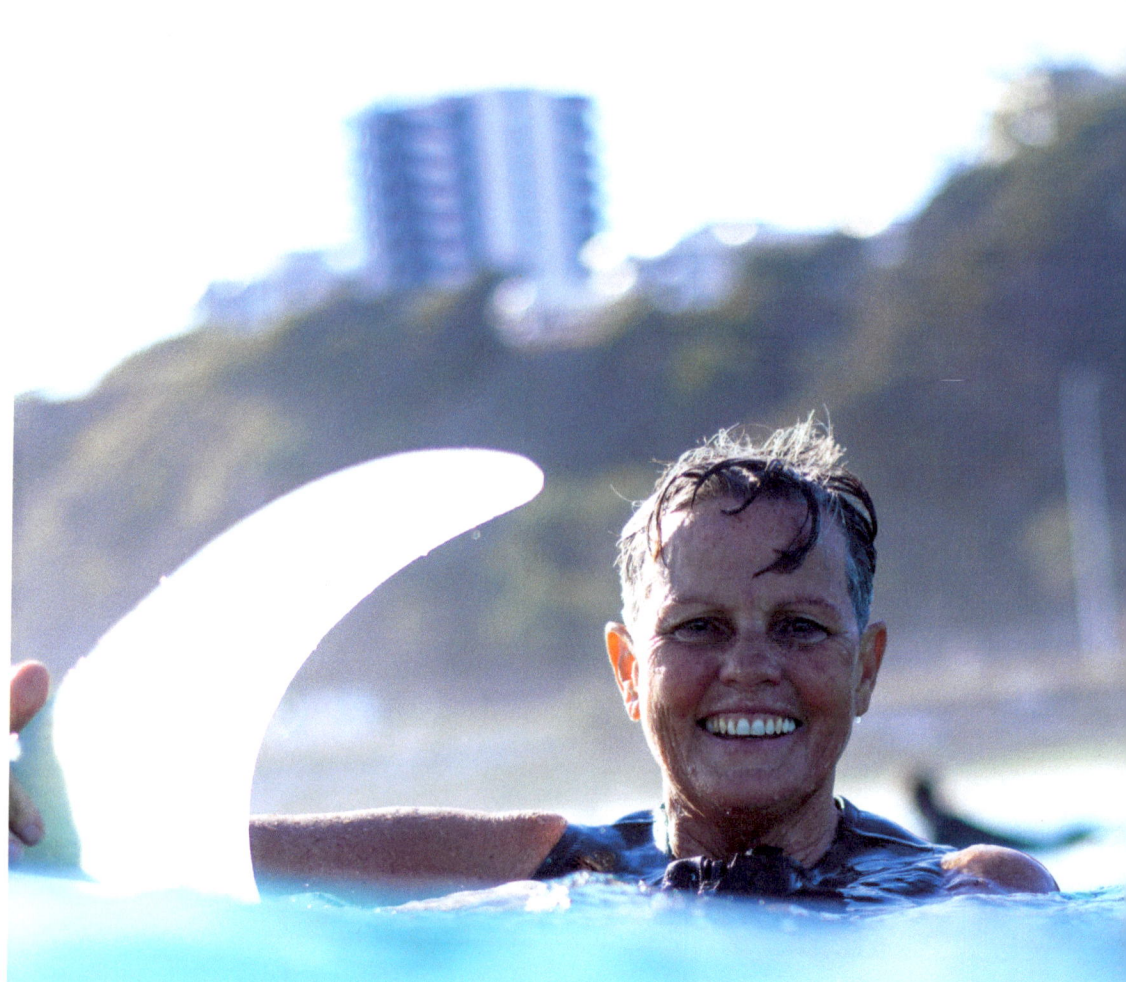

Asking for help is a power move and essential to our wellbeing.

THE PERPETUAL STRESS LOOP

WHAT IS IT?

The stress loop occurs when something or someone triggers us, and we fight in flight. Cortisol rises, we shrug our shoulders, pinch our vagus nerve, and our body goes out of balance. When we're in that place, it's easy to stay looping because when we're stressed, the stress of being stressed keeps us looping.

Naturopathically, if we can break one point on that loop, we can stop looping and move forward. That's the challenge. We need to recognise, feel, and see how our bodies react. Start by doing even one of these steps to break the perpetual stress loop. Even better, some of these practices can become habits and prevent the body from looping in the first place.

THE STRESS RESPONSES

FIGHT:

The body is on high alert. Tight, strong, and ready to depend on itself against the imposing threat of danger.

FLIGHT:

We are restless and ready to run. Feeling trapped, our heart races, and our breathing is short and sharp. We're ready to get out of there.

FREEZE:

Our body 'plays dead' during extreme stress as a physical strategy. However, it also stops us from taking self-preservation or action. Like the "deer in the headlights", we can get frozen in place, physically stiff.

FLOP:

We want to flee what is stressing us out, but our body goes limp. Our muscles go floppy. This is an automatic response by our body to help reduce physical pain from what is happening to us.

Stress and Fear only exist in the Future. Never in the Present.

THE STAGES OF THE PERPETUAL STRESS LOOP

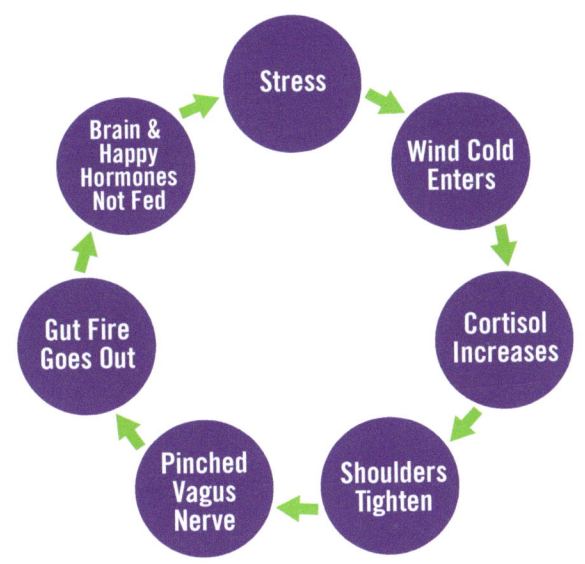

Wind Cold Enters

Wind is said to rattle our constitution and is seen as the root of many diseases in Traditional Chinese Medicine. Just like it moves and disturbs the leaves and branches of a tree, it does the same to our body systems.

After a long workday, we start to notice we're feeling tired and tight in the shoulders, neck, and back of the head. When we tax our adrenal glands, it starts to show in the neck and shoulders. We think we have poor posture from sitting at our desks or similar positions, which can be part of the problem. However, my experience in the clinic has shown that it can also be a sign of sneaky wind imbalance.

Some ways to dispel wind from our bodies are with spices like black pepper, ginger, and cinnamon. As an aromatherapist, any massage oil I make to help aching neck and shoulders always contains spice essential oils. Increasing the spice foods in our diet, along with garlic and green onion, is also very useful. The goal is to notice the aches in our neck and shoulders, listen to our body and understand that it's trying to tell that we are burning the candle at both ends and self-care is needed.

Sauna or magnesium salt baths are two of my favourite ways of warming the body. As the skin absorbs magnesium during a bath, it helps muscle relaxation and eases tension, making it an excellent remedy for a tired body. Magnesium also plays a crucial role in regulating neurotransmitters, helping reduce stress and bring a sense of calm and relaxation. A warm magnesium salt bath before bed also helps improve our sleep quality, as magnesium helps regulate melatonin production, which is essential for a restful night's sleep.

Cortisol Increases

The stress hormone cortisol is good for us when it's in balance. It's part of what gives us the energy to get out of bed every day. The problem is when we are stressing about things consistently, we're not getting those breaks, and we are not getting the recovery time that helps us bring the hormones back into balance. It can dampen the digestive system and cause food to stew instead of digest. This influences our gut and can stop our brain and gut from talking to each other. What do I mean? If the fire has gone out in our gut and food is stewing, we can't take up nutrients, especially the amino acids in foods that are needed to turn on our happy hormones. Remember, we can get stressed about being stressed and get on this perpetual loop. We need to be able to bring that cortisol back into balance. This can be done with adaptogens, which we'll get to later in the book.

The Shoulders Tighten

When we're under stress and our cortisol is too high we pull or shrug our shoulders up to our ears. Do it right now as you are reading this. We know the feeling when we get tight on those points on the top of his shoulders. When that happens, that's when we pinch the vagus nerve. This simplifies and makes it easier to understand what's happening and act.

Pinched Vagus Nerve

The vagus nerve is a vital piece of the wellbeing puzzle. Think of it like our body's secret weapon, quietly working behind the scenes to keep everything in check. This nerve is like a super-highway, linking up our brain with key organs like our heart, lungs, stomach, and gut. Yes, our gut.

The vagus nerve is one of the longest in our body, stretching from our brain down to our belly. Its name, 'vagus', means 'wandering' in Latin as it winds its way through our body.

This superhighway constantly sends messages back and forth between our brain and our organs. It's like a nonstop conversation, making sure everything from our heart rate to our digestion stays on track.

When it comes to our heart, the vagus nerve is the boss. It steps in to slow down our heart rate when it's racing, returning it to a steady rhythm when we're all worked up. The vagus nerve also plays a crucial role in digestion, helping to move food through our digestive tract, stimulate the release of stomach acid and digestive enzymes, and regulate nutrient absorption.

Remember that we are emotional beings, so the vagus nerve isn't just about the physical. It's also deeply connected to our emotions. Ever get that feeling of butterflies in your stomach when you're feeling when nervous? That's the vagus nerve at work, responding to our emotions and influencing our gut function. When feeling stressed, anxious, or just plain frazzled, activating the vagus nerve can help calm our nerves and bring us back to the centre. It's like a built-in stress-relief system, helping to calm our nervous system and promote relaxation. It's all about finding balance.

Taking slow, deep breaths, getting moving with gentle exercise like walking, Qi Gong, Tai Chi, yoga, and carving out moments of calm throughout our day can all help boost our vagal tone and support our overall wellbeing.

THE PERPETUAL STRESS LOOP

Vagal tone helps us with better emotional regulation and resilience to stress. It can be influenced by various things such as deep breathing, mindfulness practices, physical exercise, and social connections. Yes, being connected others.

My favourite breathing technique to help relax the vagus nerve is the two sniffs, and a long exhale. This simple breathing technique is like a gentle massage for our vagus nerve, soothing it into blissful relaxation. With each inhale through the nose, we activate our body's calming response, signalling to our brain that it's time to chill out. As we release that long exhale, we give our vagus nerve a little love tap, encouraging it to work magic and boost vagal tone. It's amazing how something as basic as breathing can profoundly impact our wellbeing, helping to ease stress, promote relaxation, and support our overall health. When we feel frazzled, notice, take a moment to pause, take two sniffs in, and let out a slow, steady breath—it's like hitting the reset button for our nervous system.

> **Something as basic as breathing can profoundly impact our wellbeing, helping to ease stress, promote relaxation, and support our overall health.**

Humming, chanting, or singing are also excellent for activating and stimulating the vagus nerve, supporting relaxation, and reducing stress. When we make deep, resonant sounds like "mmm" or "om," vibrations are created within our chest cavity. These vibrations travel through the vagus nerve, triggering a response that helps lower heart rate, blood pressure, and cortisol levels. This helps bring a state of calmness and relaxation. Regular practice of humming helps stress management and improves our overall wellbeing by bringing in a sense of inner peace and emotional balance. To hum is simple and powerful; we can do it quickly and quietly in a stressful situation. Yes, we can do it even quietly at work. It's an effective way to build relaxation and reduce the effects of chronic stress on both our mind and body.

Remember, our bodies are complex. We are not one body system—we are a body of body systems. Everything is interconnected, and the vagus nerve plays a central role in keeping everything running smoothly. By nurturing this vital neural highway, we're not just improving our physical health but also nurturing our emotional wellbeing.

> *Humming brings a sense of inner peace and emotional balance*

The Gut Fire Goes Out

As a naturopath, I see the gut as like a big slow cooker, a hot pot. It is hot and cooks anything added to it. Now picture tipping in a jug of ice-cold water. What does it do? It makes the cold and damp and puts the fire out and whatever we had in there that what was cooking, is now "stewing or broiling".

Consider cooking a steak on the grill if you need a visual. If the grill is not hot enough yet and we place the meat on it, the juices start to leach out of the meat and the meat starts to stew and broil. This same process happens in our gut.

Along comes stress. That cascade of events allows us to stand, fight, or get out of there. Our non-essential body processes, like digestion, sexual desire, and reproduction, are shut down. Then, the body says we are in survival mode; let's stay alive and deal with the rest later. It's why our libido is one of the first things to leave us when we are under stress. The body is focusing all its energy on the muscles and brain.

THE PERPETUAL STRESS LOOP

Whether we like it or not, we are emotional beings, and our physical bodies respond to our emotions constantly. Life is a constant dance, and we can become stuck in a loop with one of these areas off balance, which can keep feeding the other.

> **Our gut chemistry can help ease stress, depression and anxiety, but it can also feed it.**

This is why someone can eat a raw, vegan, paleo, keto, whole-food diet but still have a very out-of-balance body. Healthy food meets a stress-affected gut, and the food stews instead of digesting the nutrients. This, in turn, affects our brain. Our gut chemistry can help ease stress, depression and anxiety, but it can also feed it. We stay in the perpetual stress loop.

"All disease begins in the gut."

HIPPOCRATES

The Brain and Happy Hormones Aren't Fed

Think of our brain as a big lump of omega-3 fat with an electrical system running through it. It's approximately 60% fat and 40% water, proteins and carbohydrates, which are essential to a healthy brain function.

Our brain functions best when fed with essential nutrients, particularly omega-3 fatty acids, which are crucial in turning on neurotransmitters associated with our feelings of happiness. Eating a diet rich in nutrients, such as good fats, is essential for maintaining our mental wellbeing. Including omega-3-rich foods in our diet is necessary. Flaxseed oil is my favourite, and it is an excellent source of omega-3. I recommended adding flaxseed oil on salads or two teaspoons to my nutritional smoothies daily. Eating omega-3-rich snacks like walnuts and pumpkin seeds into our daily routine can also help our mental health. Just ensure they are consumed in their raw form close to nature to preserve the integrity of the omega-3 fatty acids. An important note is that Omega 3 essential fatty acids are destroyed with heat and light, so don't cook them and store them in the refrigerator. We'll talk more about this in the Food chapter of this book.

The stress cycle repeats if our body and brain are not fed properly. We keep looping and stay out of balance. The most common areas of health we see this influencing first are sleep, energy, moods, and weight.

Amino acids play a crucial role in turning on the release of happy hormones in the brain. They are the essential building blocks of protein. They can stimulate the production and release of neurotransmitters, such as serotonin, dopamine, and endorphins, often called our 'happy hormones'. When amino acids are eaten through a balanced diet, they are broken down and used by the body to synthesise these neurotransmitters. For example, the amino acid tryptophan is converted into serotonin, which is responsible for regulating mood, sleep, and appetite. The amino acid tyrosine is transformed into dopamine, the neurotransmitter associated with pleasure and reward. Eating foods rich in essential amino acids provides the amino acids to help feed our overall wellbeing and happiness.

Sesame seeds, pumpkin seeds, almonds, cheese, soybeans (edamame), nuts, lean grass-fed meats, fish, eggs, quinoa, cottage cheese, and Greek yoghurt are an excellent place to start when ensuring you get a variety of essential amino acids.

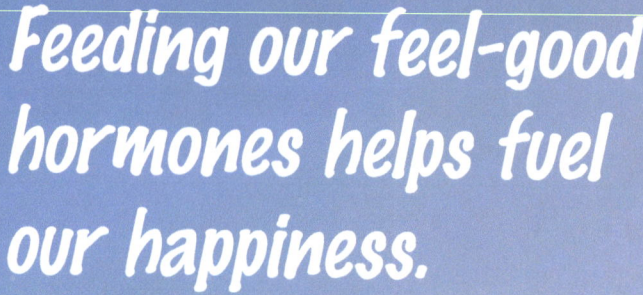

Feeding our feel-good hormones helps fuel our happiness.

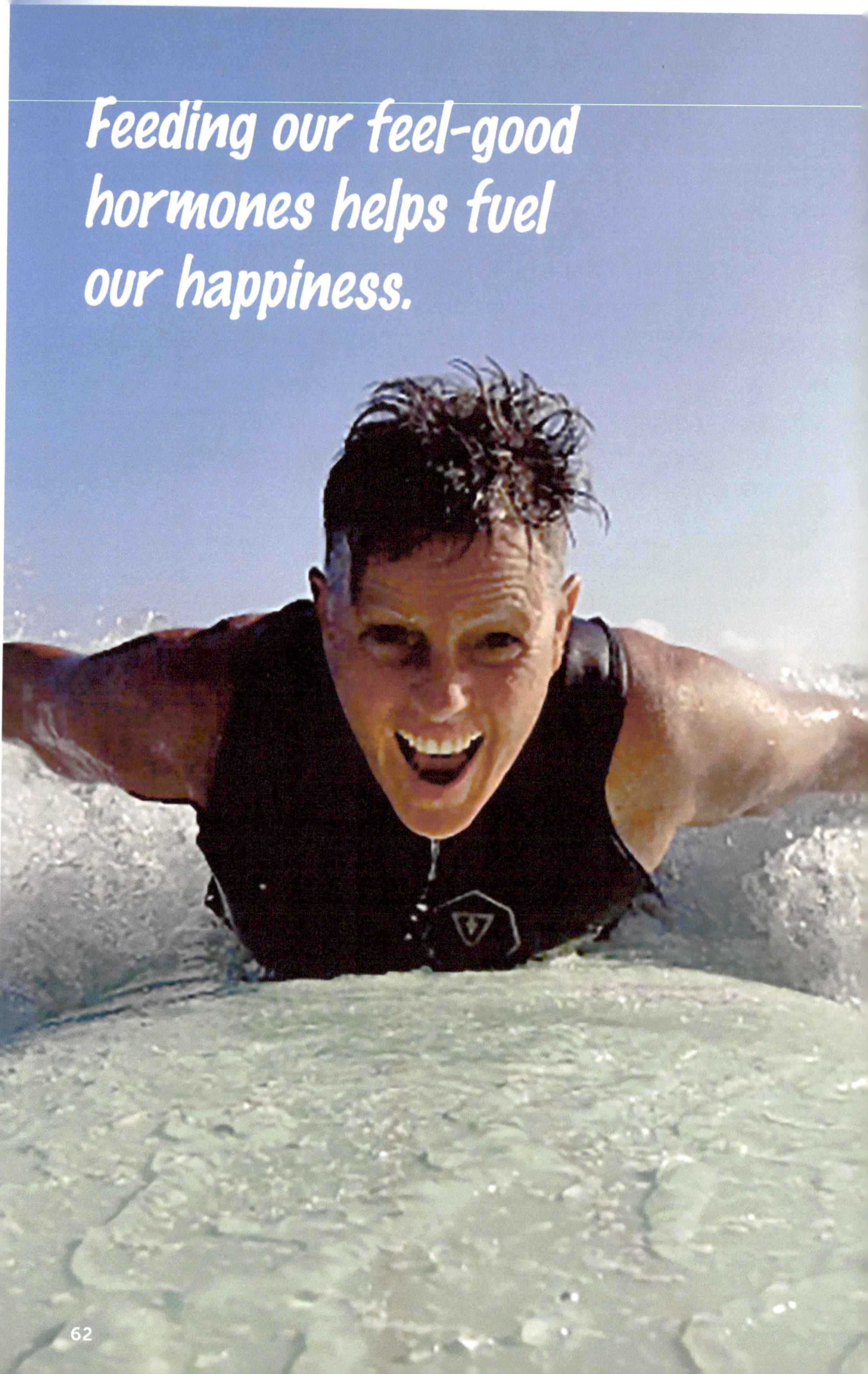

The BAM

TO BREAK THE STRESS LOOP

The Bare Arse Minimum (BAM) approach nurtures the body, moving away from adrenal survival mode through the practice of good food, good rest, and good play.

Physical and emotional stress demands can deeply deplete our adrenal glands, which are seen as reservoirs of life energy or Qi in Traditional Chinese Medicine.

THE BAM TO BREAK THE STRESS LOOP

Unlike quick-fix solutions, which I am not a fan of, replenishing adrenal health requires consistent investment in these basics. Like managing a bank account, adrenal survival hinges on daily balance. Energy is spent and banked regularly. Without regular deposits, there is nothing left to draw upon. Making balance our priority is not a sign of weakness; it is crucial for thriving without burning out. Success in our professional and personal lives depends on maintaining healthy and adaptable adrenal health.

> **It's not about slowing down or going without the things we love. It's living in a way that feeds us, instead of sucking the life from us.**

What's great is the BAM approach isn't about slowing down or going without the things we love. It's about living in a way that life feeds us energy instead of sucking the life from us.

MAKING THE TIME FOR GREAT HEALTH

It is so important to prioritise good food, good rest, and good play in our daily lives. Mindfully integrating these practices into our busy schedules is essential for overall wellbeing. Simply hitting the gym sporadically or taking occasional breaks won't work. Consistent lifestyle changes, no matter how small, are necessary for lasting benefits.

> **It is so important to prioritise good food, good rest, and good play in our daily lives.**

Let's be honest and talk about managing our time in a way that supports our actual wellbeing. Many of us are pros at juggling our work commitments, and it's time to stop treating our work and personal lives like two separate entities Everything we do contributes to our overall life, and nowadays, the line between work and personal time isn't as clear-cut as it used to be. I merge my work and personal schedules into one "life diary". I block out the times for all my family and life commitments, including things like "date night" first. Putting everything into one schedule, particularly our non-negotiables first, can free up our brain, and we gain a clearer picture of what needs to be done. It can be easier to incorporate self-care into our daily routine. The power move is not to cancel our self-care appointments because we are busy. Why mention that? Because I know it's something most people need to sort out. We need to make our health a priority first. It's not selfish. It's self-preservation.

Making our health our priority is not selfish its self-preservation.

Once we have all our business meetings, social commitments, and self-care in our diary, it's also a place to schedule some quiet time alone for reflection and dreaming. Have you ever noticed how we hardly ever sit and think these days? Our minds are constantly buzzing with activity, "doing" instead of "being". Taking time to pause and reflect is crucial for avoiding burnout. Instead of bouncing from one task to the next, set aside ten minutes daily to focus on quiet time.

Taking time to pause and reflect is crucial for avoiding burnout.

Dr. Andrew Huberman created the term NSDR, or Non-Sleep Deep Rest. The concept brings a revolutionary approach to improving rest and rejuvenation without requiring traditional sleep. This technique focuses on achieving deep restorative states through specific relaxation practices like meditation and controlled breathing exercises. By tapping into the body's natural ability to deeply relax while remaining awake, we can experience profound physiological and psychological benefits, including reduced stress, improved cognitive function, and enhanced overall wellbeing. If we have ever been to a yoga session, the ten-minute relaxation at the end, the Shavasana, is a form of NSDR and is a restful and rejuvenating yoga posture. It literally translates as 'corpse pose' and involves lying face-up on the ground with arms and legs naturally extended and eyes gently closed. I find it deliciously relaxing.

Here are a few ways to practice NSDR:

1. Mindfulness and meditation techniques can help calm the mind and bring deep relaxation. Find a quiet and comfortable space, focus on your breath, and let go of any tension or stress in your body. Even five minutes of meditation can help achieve NSDR.

2. Deep breathing techniques, such as diaphragmatic (belly) or box breathing, can help activate our body's relaxation response. Box breathing is a relaxation technique involving breathing in, holding, breathing out, and holding again in equal counts, generally four. Focusing on our breath and taking slow, deep belly breaths can reduce stress and promote NSDR.

3. Guided visualisation, or Yoga Nidra, involves using our imagination to create soothing and calming mental images. We close our eyes, imagine ourselves in a peaceful and serene environment, and engage all our senses in this visualisation. This can help relax our mind and body, promoting NSDR. My wife Alice has the perfect voice for guided visualisation and has recorded some you can listen to for free. Check out the resource list at the back of this book.

4. Shavasana, as I mentioned at the end of a yoga session, can help induce a state of NSDR.

Deep rest is vital for our overall wellbeing, and scheduling time for relaxation and rejuvenation. Play with different techniques and find what works best to help achieve a non-sleep deep rest.

> Deep rest is vital for our overall wellbeing, and scheduling time for relaxation and rejuvenation.

I am a huge Einstein fan. He was known to benefit from periods of rest while awake, which allowed him to engage in what he called "combinatory play" or creative thinking. Einstein often took breaks during his work to play the violin or sail, which allowed his mind to wander and make connections between seemingly unrelated ideas. These periods of restful wakefulness allowed him to approach problems from new perspectives and ultimately contributed to his ground-breaking scientific discoveries.

Whether for 10 minutes or an hour, this form of rest brings better results and leaves us feeling more in control and relaxed.

In my schedule, I lock in everything from business appointments and deadlines to quality time with friends and family and self-care activities like massages, quiet time, meals, playing my ukulele and exercise. In the past, I remember sitting at my desk, on edge with the phone tucked under my ear, checking voicemails while I was responding to an email, and an SMS arrived! It was all going on at once. Most people can only focus on something for a few minutes before the phone rings, an email arrives, or someone drops by the desk to 'ask a quick question'. We're at risk of becoming a workforce that can't think, plan, and manage strategic goals because we're so used to reacting to interruptions. We need to set rules about how we work and get technology working for us rather than us working for it.

> **We're at risk of becoming a workforce that can't think, plan, and manage strategic goals because we're so used to reacting to interruptions.**

Today I have NO notifications on anything. Email, text, socials, App's, nothing. I set an alarm when I am expecting a call or a meeting. I choose to check my emails once or twice a day rather than every time a new one pops into the inbox. The freedom and peace I have from not being distracted endlessly is bliss. I know many people who claim that they can multitask or are too busy to do just one thing at a time. But it's not about slowing down; it's about becoming more productive, effective and less stressed.

When we become distracted from a task, it typically takes around 15 minutes to regain complete focus and return to our previous level of productivity. It's known as "task-switching" or "attention residue" and occurs because our brains need time to transition back to the original task after being interrupted. By the way, every distraction is equal. Even a brief distraction can disrupt our concentration and cause our attention to wander, making it challenging to resume work efficiently. During this transition period, our brains must return to the centre and re-establish the focus and momentum necessary to continue. Minimising distractions and staying focused on one task at a time can significantly help us to "get shit done" and reduce stress.

By the way, I have a "go fast" ADHD brain, and I have had to work hard to find strategies like these to keep me focused.

I understand that scheduling personal time might feel like you're killing spontaneity. But it is time to be honest with yourself. How is not scheduling time for yourself working out? If you're not finding time for spontaneity, it's time to schedule some! Planned spontaneity works to break habits and patterns.

Many of us feel like we never have time for ourselves, but that's because we haven't made it a priority. Think about all the things we make time for in our life. If taking care of ourselves isn't high on our list of priorities, it's time to change that. We can't just decide to make time for ourselves; we must schedule it and stick to the schedule. So, grab the new 'life' diary and start locking in some self-care time.

If we don't have time or mindset to play, it's time to Plan Some Spontaneity!

SELF-CARE

Self-care is often mistakenly seen as indulgences like spa days or vacations, but it's true value lies in the daily habits and choices that sustain our wellbeing. It includes all the small activities we do consistently, such as prioritising adequate sleep, regular exercise, eating close to nature 80% of the time, nurturing a positive mindset, noticing what we feed our minds, who we hang out with, and so on. These daily rituals are the foundation of self-care because they directly influence physical health, mental resilience, and emotional balance.

> **True value lies in the daily habits and choices that sustain our wellbeing.**

For instance, getting enough sleep allows our bodies to repair and recharge, while regular exercise improves physical fitness, boosts mood, and reduces stress. Mindful eating ensures we nourish our bodies with the necessary nutrients, supporting overall vitality. Managing our mindset involves practices like meditation, gratitude, or journaling, which help build resilience and emotional wellbeing through life's challenges. Who we spend our time with and what we listen to and feed our minds with have us in a positive, uplifting environment or not. Our life force, our Qi, depends on us spending and refilling the health bank account daily. Not just periodically. I meet many people who think it is just having a regular spa day or massage, and it's far from that. Integrating self-care into our daily routines empowers us to make sustainable choices that bring us long-term health and happiness. It goes beyond the occasional luxury to embody a lifestyle of preventative holistic wellbeing.

> **Integrating self-care into our daily routines empowers us to make sustainable choices that bring us long-term health and happiness.**

Be a self-care rebel.

Self-care
is not a Luxury
it's a Necessity
for our Wellbeing.

GOOD FOOD BAM

Many of us are lucky to have plenty of food in the Western world. We don't usually worry about where our next meal will come from. But this abundance has made us forget that food is fuel for our bodies. We eat to give our bodies the energy and materials they need to work, grow, and stay healthy.

For many people, though, food is more about enjoying tasty treats or eating for reasons that don't involve staying healthy. We might snack without thinking, eat when feeling down, or feast when catching up with friends even though we're not hungry. Sometimes, we even fill up on stuff that we know isn't good for us. Instead of treating food as something that helps us, we end up hurting ourselves with it.

It's weird when we think about it. Some parts of the world struggle to get enough food to eat, while others have so much that it's causing health problems like obesity and diseases related to being overweight.

We need to get serious about how we think about food. What we eat most of the time affects our body and health. We often focus on how our bodies look from the outside but forget what's happening inside at the minor level. But whether we eat too much or too little, it can harm our bodies, and eventually, we'll feel the consequences.

What if instead of obsessing over diets or using food to comfort ourselves, we saw food as the fuel our bodies need to function well? Our bodies are incredible machines. Much of what keeps our bodies running smoothly happens without us even realising it. We might overlook the daily work our bodies do to keep us healthy until something goes wrong.

If we start thinking of food as fuel, we can make better choices about what we eat. It's about prioritising our health and making healthy choices 80% of the time. Why not 100%? 100% of nothing is nothing. Striving for 100%, going off track and giving up means we achieve nothing.

100% of Nothing is Nothing.

Eat Close to Nature 80% of the time and 80% of our health works.

THE FOOD PYRAMID IS REALLY SQUARE

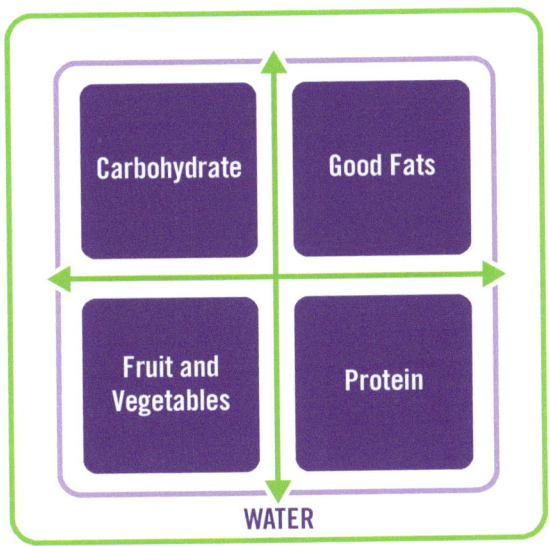

Many of us are familiar with the food pyramid, a visual guide often taught in schools, telling us the right foods to eat for good health. However, few people realise that this dietary guideline, deemed ideal by the United States Department of Agriculture (USDA), is crafted in collaboration with powerful industry groups shaping the standard Western diet. It's no coincidence that entities like the National Dairy Council, United Fresh Fruit and Vegetable Association, Soft Drink Association, American Meat Institute, National Cattlemen's Beef Association, and Wheat Foods Council exert considerable influence over the pyramid's recommendations.

Despite the involvement of nutrition experts, I worry about whose interests these guidelines genuinely serve. According to the Harvard School of Public Health, the selection process for panelists responsible for these recommendations is heavily influenced by lobbying efforts from industry organisations. The repercussions of such dietary advice are increasingly evident in soaring rates of chronic illnesses like heart disease, diabetes, obesity, and related health issues within Western populations.

Travelling the world, I see traditional Asian and European diets are closer to their natural state. These diets, known for their cleanliness and balance, have traditionally had lower incidences of lifestyle-related diseases than their Western counterparts. However, as Westernised diets and fast foods penetrate the world, these once-distinct health advantages are gradually eroding. I see in my travels how the shift towards processed and convenience crap foods is contributing to a rise in diet-related health challenges rarely seen there before and so common in the West.

> **The secret is to eat foods as close to their natural state as possible.**

The secret is to eat foods as close to their natural state as possible. So, if we're going to eat grains, eat them unrefined; if we're going to eat meat, go grass-fed and organic; and if we're going to cook vegetables, lightly steam them with the lid on the pot so that we reduce the loss of nutrients through cooking. Eating this way is simple, and that's part of the problem; it's so simple that it gets missed. If things are easy to do, they are also easy not to do.

If things are easy to do, they are also easy not to do.

WATER BAM

My food pyramid is a square in which the foods we should be eating are surrounded by the number one element our bodies need – water. Our bodies are mostly water – about 60-70%. That means our muscles, blood, and even bones contain a lot of water. It makes sense why people keep telling us to drink more water, right?

Water is super important for our bodies. It helps keep us hydrated, especially our brains. When we don't drink enough water, our brain feels it first, which can mess with our thinking. Water also helps flush out the bad stuff from our bodies, like when we're stressed and our bodies release acidic wastes.

> **When we don't drink enough water, our brain feels it first, which can mess with our thinking.**

How much water do we need? I recommend drinking about 33 millilitres per kilo of filtered water's desired body weight daily. This is what an active person needs just to stay hydrated. Why filtered? Regular water can have chemicals like chlorine or bacteria that aren't good for us. Let me be clear, though: If you don't have access to filtered water, still drink water. Don't use that as an excuse for not drinking.

People say to me, Jen, I can't drink that much water, yet they drink that much liquid in all the unhealthy drinks. Before I learned the importance of water, I never did either. I taught myself by setting an alarm on my digital watch in the 1980s. Today, we have phones that make it easier to set alarms. I recommend setting an alarm hourly for each hour you are awake. For instance, if we generally wake at 6am, set an alarm for 7 am and hourly from then. Then, hit the repeat each day of the week. The alarms are set, and it makes it easy to create a new habit. Eventually, we don't need an alarm to remind us to drink a glass of water an hour. I promise our bodies will love us for setting this new habit.

When I talk about water, I mean just that – water. Even though tea, coffee, and alcoholic drinks contain water, our bodies must work harder to use it. So, it's better to stick to plain water or herbal teas, like green tea brewed for less than a minute, to get the good antioxidants and caffeine without too much dehydrating tannin. Yes, tannin is what is used to turn animal hides into leather. So, brew it for less than a minute and like herb tea, it counts as water. Think about that the next time while drinking a cup of tea.

FRUIT AND VEGETABLES BAM

Fruit and vegetables in the diet is a whole book on its own. The BAM approach, though, promotes diversity in our daily eating. The latest research indicates that incorporating a diverse range of foods into our diet is essential not just for nutrients but also for maintaining a healthy gut microbiome. Recent studies, like the American Gut Study, suggest that eating at least 30 different types of foods each week can promote microbial diversity in the gut, which helps with improved digestion, immune function, and overall wellbeing. This diversity allows for a rich ecosystem of bacteria to flourish in the gut, assisting the breakdown and absorption of nutrients, reducing inflammation and protecting against certain diseases. My wife Alice and I aim for 30 different foods every day.

> **Incorporating a diverse range of foods into our diet is essential not just for nutrients but also for maintaining a healthy gut microbiome.**

Prioritising a colourful and varied diet that includes a wide array of fruits, vegetables, whole grains, legumes, nuts, seeds, and fermented foods can be crucial in nurturing a thriving gut microbiome and promoting optimal health. More on that later in the book.

I get asked all the time if organic is better. Bottom line is no. Daily stress, worry and overwork or overwhelm can change our body chemistry faster than bad food. It's not just what we eat. It's how our body deals with and assimilates what we eat that matters. Otherwise, we are adding yummy healthy food into a dirty (and I'm not talking poo), usually hormonally out-of-balance body. That's why we can eat clean, organic and healthy and still be dragging our butt around. Yes, stress overrides organic nutrition. It overrides everything.

While organic food is considered a healthier eating choice and is thought to be more nutritious, the reality can be different.

However, the reality can be different. While organic farming prohibits the use of synthetic pesticides, herbicides, and fertilisers, it doesn't guarantee higher nutrition. Organic produce may lack chemical residues, making them a better choice. The nutrient levels in organic foods can vary widely depending on factors like soil quality, growing conditions, and crop variety. Organic farming practices contribute to environmental sustainability and reduce chemical exposure, which is great. However, we must still manage our stress and prioritise a balanced diet and diverse food choices to ensure optimal nutrition. Just going organic isn't the answer.

I look for "close to nature" and at home "we grow food, not grass", so I know what goes into our basic vegetables. Managing our stress is our highest priority, so there will be lots of info coming up on that.

What's better, raw or cooked? A blend of both gets my naturopath tick. Remember that our gut is like a big crock pot, putting in cold raw foods constantly kills the fire in our gut. I am a bigger fan of lightly steamed than raw myself. When steaming or cooking, always use a lid to evaporate the water-soluble nutrients in the steam.

PROTEIN BAM

Animal or plant-based protein? Let's look at the BAM on both.

When considering red meat options, grass-fed game meat, like kangaroo in Australia, stands out as a superior choice for protein intake. It boasts the highest protein content and lowest saturated fat levels among all red meats. Kangaroo meat is also renowned as the richest natural source of conjugated linoleic acid (CLA), a beneficial fatty acid typically found in grass-fed animals. CLA has been linked to potential health benefits such as anti-carcinogenic and anti-diabetic properties and aiding in the reduction of obesity and atherosclerosis (high blood pressure). Choosing kangaroo meat supports protein needs and provides a healthier alternative with genuine nutritional advantages.

Fish is another excellent source of protein and healthy fats. Cold water fish, like salmon, are packed with good fats and omega-3s. Be aware that farmed fish, like salmon, are not good. Just as our body chemistry changes under stress, so does an animal's body. Choose sustainably wild caught sources only.

> **The same as our body chemistry changes when we are under stress so does an animal. Think about that when choosing your protein source.**

If we're not into meat or fish, egg whites are an excellent protein source, too. Just be sure to get "happy free-range eggs".

When it comes to dairy, go for grass-fed and organic options like yoghurt or cottage cheese. They're easier to digest and still give your body the protein and fat it needs.

As a naturopath, I see food intolerances to dairy and gluten as a gut chemistry imbalance. If you're allergic, that's different. If you're just sensitive, don't eliminate it; work to rebalance the cause behind the food intolerance, which will be in the gut.

My wife Alice and I choose to eat a plant-based diet at home. Yes, we have the occasional fish meal if we are eating out. Vegetarians have thrived for years without consuming animal products. Lentils, beans, legumes, tofu, and tempeh are wonderful sources of protein and are low-GI carbohydrates. Nuts and seeds are another solid source of protein, minerals and fat-soluble nutrients, but they're also very high in fat (68-78%). It's good fat, but it's still fat. The good oils found in nuts and seeds are easily damaged by heat, light, and oxygen, so always eat unsalted nuts and seeds directly from their shells if you can. If you cook with nuts or seeds, add them at the last moment so that the heat doesn't destroy the nutrients.

So, how much protein per day? The older I get and the further I dive into this subject, the clearer it becomes that the recommended daily allowance (RDA) of 0.8 grams per kilogram of body weight is not enough to build and sustain muscle mass as we age which is an essential part of an exercise program for promoting longevity. As a naturopath, I eat and advise clients to target a protein intake of 1.6 to 2 grams per kilogram of desired body weight (or approximately 1 gram per pound) per day.

Maintaining adequate protein intake as adults age becomes increasingly important to support overall health and wellbeing. Protein plays a crucial role in preserving muscle mass, bone density, and immune function, all of which can decline with age. Research suggests that older adults may require higher protein intake to offset age-related muscle loss (sarcopenia) and support good physical function. Promoting muscle protein synthesis and repair, eating around 100 grams of protein per day is recommended for ageing adults. This amount helps ensure that our body has an adequate supply of essential amino acids necessary for tissue maintenance and repair, as well as for supporting metabolic functions and immune response.

Elderly people who increase their protein intake are at a reduced risk of experiencing a decline in "functioning," such as dressing independently, getting out of bed, climbing stairs, and other daily activities. Retaining our lean muscle as we age is essential, and protein is the key. I plan to be strong, fit and healthy as I age, and I do the work today for that to evolve.

The BAM is to eat and live, not to let the old lady in.

> **Retaining our lean muscle as we age is essential, and protein is the key.**

A common mistake people make is thinking that a 100-gram chicken breast, for instance, is 100 grams of protein. However, 100 grams of meat does not equate to 100 grams of protein due to the varying protein content of different types of meat. Lean meats generally provide more protein per gram compared to fatty cuts, which contain higher proportions of fat alongside protein.

Some protein amounts in foods

- **Fish:** Half a salmon fillet (124g) = 30.5g protein; Cod fillet (180g) = 41g protein.
- **Shellfish:** 3-ounce (85g) serving cooked clams = 21.8g protein; 3-ounce (85g) serving of shrimp/prawns = 20.4g protein.
- **Skinless, white-meat poultry:** Half chicken breast (86g) = 26.7g protein.
- **Lean beef:** 3-ounce (85g) serving = 24.6g protein.
- **Cottage cheese:** One cup (226g) = 28g protein.
- **Greek yoghurt:** 7-ounce (200g) container = 19.9g protein.
- **Eggs:** One large egg (50g) = 6.3g protein.
- **Peanuts:** 1-ounce (28.35g) serving = 7.31g protein; 2-tablespoons (32g) smooth peanut butter = 7.2g protein.
- **Pumpkin Seeds:** 1/4 cup (29.5g) = 8.8g protein.
- **Lentils:** One cup = 18g protein.
- **Chickpeas:** One cup = 15g protein
- **Black beans:** One cup = 15g protein.
- **Tofu:** 1/2 cup = 20g protein.
- **Edamame:** One cup (shelled) = 17g protein.
- **Hemp seeds:** 3-tablespoons = 10g protein.
- **Quinoa:** One cup (cooked) = 8g protein.
- **Chia seeds:** 2-tablespoons = 6g protein.
- **Spinach:** One cup (cooked) = 5g protein.
- **Almonds:** 1/4 cup = 6g protein.
- **Pistachios:** 1-ounce (28.35g) = 5.73g protein.
- **Cashews:** 1-ounce (28.35g) = 4.34g protein.

Protein Pacing

What is it? Protein pacing spreads our protein intake evenly throughout the day to improve muscle protein synthesis and overall health benefits. Eating moderate amounts of protein consistently across meals and snacks can better support muscle repair, growth, and maintenance. This approach helps the body utilise protein efficiently, promotes satiety, and helps regulate our appetite, potentially aiding in weight wellness.

> **Eating moderate amounts of protein consistently across meals and snacks can better support muscle repair, growth, and maintenance.**

Protein pacing is not just for athletes. Most commonly, people are light on protein in the morning and tend to have their larger and more protein-dense meal in the evening. Research suggests that spreading our protein intake across the day may be more beneficial than eating large amounts in a single meal, as it provides a steady supply of amino acids necessary for physiological functions.

The Bedtime Belly Buster (BBB)

What is the BBB? It is a low-calorie protein snack eaten 30 to 60 minutes before bed that may increase our metabolic rate and even reduce early morning hunger. Late-night snacking is often blamed for weight gain. However, researchers suggest that the nutritional quality of a bedtime snack determines its impact on our waistline. Many people choose less healthy options like ice cream and chips to satisfy late-night cravings mindlessly in front of the TV.

Research shows that protein-rich diets can help weight loss while preserving muscle mass. The Health, Aging, and Body Composition (Health ABC) Study showed that older adults eating higher amounts of dietary protein experienced a 40% reduction in lean muscle mass loss compared to those with lower protein intakes. The protein quality is crucial; sources containing high levels of branched-chain amino acids are particularly effective in promoting muscle growth and supporting weight maintenance.

A 40-gram serving of protein equates to approximately 180 grams (6 ounces) of steak or chicken breast, and we are not just getting the protein element from the food. We are getting the extra calories from not just the protein of the meat. Not everyone wants to eat 40 grams of protein before sleeping, but if I was focused on weight loss, consuming even 20 grams of protein 30-60 minutes before bedtime may help boost my metabolism. People aiming to increase muscle mass and strength can benefit from eating 40 grams of protein before bed.

With protein pacing in mind, this can be a way to help us get our protein in for the day. I choose to use a high-quality whey protein concentrate from grass-fed New Zealand happy cows for my BBB, and I pair it with a dose of adaptogens within 30 minutes of my sleep. Why? I want to tap into multiple benefits to help my sleep as well.

Eat and live to NOT let the Old Lady in.

GOOD CARBS BAM

Remember when we made glue out of white flour and water at school? Remember how it smelt after a few hours and set like cement when we used it? Well, that same cement-like action happens inside our bodies whenever we eat white bread, pasta and rice. After it has been in there for a while, it becomes foul, sticking to the walls of our bowels and sucking the life out of us. I call it 'bum glue'.

It is wise to eat whole grains that retain their wheat germ, such as whole wheat bread, pasta, and brown rice. The wheat germ is where most nutrients reside, making whole grains a nutritional powerhouse. Equally, refined and processed grains, like white bread, pasta, and rice, lack wheat germ and are typically stripped of essential nutrients during processing. These refined grains are acid-forming, primarily due to their high phosphorous content, and can lead to gastrointestinal issues such as bloating and discomfort.

> **The wheat germ is where most nutrients reside, making whole grains a nutritional powerhouse.**

Choosing refined grains in the form of flour can pose challenges to gut health, brain function, and joint health. Refined grains are rich in phytates, acidic compounds that bind minerals in the intestinal tract, preventing their absorption and leaving their excretion from the body unused. Imagine eating a 'healthy' meat and salad sandwich on white bread for lunch, which can result in the rapid loss of water-soluble nutrients from the body. A water-soluble nutrient that gets lost easily is chromium. Chromium is needed to balance blood sugar levels. So, that white bread sandwich could be spiking our insulin level and dropping our energy an hour or two later. Choosing whole grains over refined options can ensure optimal nutrient intake and support overall health and wellbeing.

GOOD FOOD BAM

My gorgeous friend and Metabolic Nutritionist, Lochi Horner, calls carbohydrates the "intensity macro". Good carbs play a crucial role in fueling our bodies for physical activity. The amount of carbs we need relates closely to our exercise intensity. When engaging in high-intensity workouts or endurance activities, carbohydrates provide the primary energy source, helping to sustain performance and prevent fatigue. In contrast, lower-intensity exercises or sedentary lifestyles require fewer carbs. Eating carbs with activity levels in mind can effectively manage energy levels, maintain healthy body composition, and promote long-term fitness and wellbeing.

> **If we did nothing other than replace white grains with wholemeal or brown alternatives in our diet, our basic level of health would increase dramatically.**

If we did nothing other than replace white grains with wholemeal or brown alternatives in our diet, our basic level of health would increase dramatically. Working out which carbohydrates to eat is easy; remember to eat close to nature, unrefined brown grains (brown rice, buckwheat, pasta, and bread).

By the way, I love pasta, and I love that today we can buy pasta made from red lentils, edamame, and a range of beans or pulses, so it is even easier to get the added protein in what would generally be a carb-loaded meal like pasta.

Don't Eat "Bum Glue".

> *Carbohydrates are the "intensity macro". The amount of carbs we need correlates with the intensity of our exercise.*
>
> — LOCHI HORNER

GOOD FATS BAM

Omega-3, omega-6, and omega-9 are essential fatty acids (EFAs) that play crucial roles in maintaining overall health but differ in their structures and functions. Omega-3 fatty acids, found abundantly in fatty fish like salmon and, flaxseeds and chia seeds, are renowned for their anti-inflammatory properties and are vital for brain and heart health and for reducing the risk of chronic diseases.

Omega-6 fatty acids, prevalent in vegetable oils like sunflower, safflower, and soybean, are also essential but, in excess, can promote inflammation. That is why maintaining a proper balance between omega-3 and omega-6 intake is key.

Omega-9 fatty acids, found in olive oil, avocados, and nuts, are not considered essential as the body can produce them. However, they still offer substantial health benefits, including supporting heart health and reducing inflammation.

To differentiate between them, remember that omega-3 fatty acids are typically associated with cold-water fatty fish, omega-6 fatty acids are commonly found in vegetable oils, and omega-9 fatty acids are prevalent in sources like olive oil and avocados.

> **When cooking with oils, choose those with a high smoking point. It is crucial for maintaining the oil's integrity and nutritional benefits at higher temperatures.**

When cooking with oils, choose those with a high smoking point. It is crucial for maintaining the oil's integrity and nutritional benefits at higher temperatures. Three of the best oils known for their high smoking points are avocado oil, olive oil, and organic peanut oil. Avocado oil boasts a smoking point of around 270°C (520°F), making it ideal for searing, frying, and sautéing. Olive oil has its smoke point at approximately 240°C (465°F), remains stable under medium to high heat, and is suitable for various cooking methods. Organic peanut oil, with a smoking point reaching about 232°C (450°F), is valued for deep frying and stir-frying due to its heat tolerance and neutral flavour profile.

One of the best books I have ever read on fats is 'Fats That Heal, Fats That Kill', by Udo Erasmus. In basic terms, he explains the nutritional differences between lifeless, refined, processed oils and cold-pressed oils that are full of nutrients. Most of the oils in the supermarket have been overheated in processing and are now rancid; margarines are even worse. When vegetable fats are overheated, they are transformed into trans fatty acids, the nastiest of all foods we can put into our bodies. In 2003, the US Government advised the creators of the food pyramid to revise it to encourage the eating of omega-essential fatty acids and the elimination of trans fatty acids from people's diets on the basis that omega-3 fatty acids may reduce the risk of coronary heart disease (CHD), while trans fatty acids may increase the risk of CHD. Sadly, the standard Western diet is still too low in good fats today.

Avocado, kangaroo, and cold-water fish are all good sources of good fats (try to avoid tinned fish, though, because it has been exposed to extreme heat during the cooking process, which makes the good fats less good). I eat avocado, nuts, and seeds and consume organic flax seed oil and extra virgin olive oils daily. I add them to salads or protein shakes to ensure I get my necessary quota of essential fatty acids.

> **Avocado, kangaroo, and cold-water fish are all good sources of good fats.**

To sum up the BAM on fats, here is a visual. Imagine that all fats are like a long chain and at every link of that chain, there is a hydrogen atom or not. Think about the fat on the side of a steak: solid, white and oh-so-delicious when cooked. It's the same as the cheese that we eat. They are solid at room temperature, and that's saturated fat. The word saturated is used to describe how the links to their chain are saturated with a hydrogen atom at each link. It's an easy visual. So now, imagine that when we eat meats and dairy, that saturated "fat" stays solid like that inside our body.

Vegetable, nut, and seed oils are typically liquid at room temperature, and the chain links are not saturated with hydrogen atoms. Some links have no hydrogen atoms, so they stay liquid. They also stay inside our bodies. We need the balance of good Omega 3, 6, and 9 oils to help balance the hard saturated fats to help prevent them from clogging our bodies. I hope that visual helps, as the impact of not being balanced is very real on our health.

BUTTER BAM

A lot has been said about butter and margarine over the years, so how do we know which is best for our health?

What is butter?

Butter begins its journey as cream, which is then churned. The cream is vigorously shaken until the milk fat, known as butter, forms and separates from the liquid part, called buttermilk. The butter is churned more until it achieves the perfect consistency for packaging.

As a fat-rich delight, butter is recognised as a high-calorie treat. Just one tablespoon of butter, weighing about 14 grams, packs around 100 calories, like the energy found in a medium-sized banana, providing 89 calories.

Loaded with essential vitamins like A, D, E, B12, and K2, butter brings valuable nutrition.

Loaded with essential vitamins like A, D, E, B12, and K2, butter brings valuable nutrition. However, it's calorie-dense. If eating butter, choose butter sourced from grass-fed cows. Yes, close to nature.

I have to talk about the supposed healthy ratings system for fats like butter and margarine. The Heart Foundation started the Tick program in 1959, with margarine makers among its earliest adopters. The Foundation openly acknowledged receiving unrestricted grants from three pharmaceutical giants — Sanofi, Astra Zeneca, and Amgen. Brands paid for the privilege of branding products with the Heart Foundation Tick, which contributed to a heightened awareness of "healthy foods" in Australian markets despite the occasional controversy over specific endorsements. To earn the Tick, packaged foods had to show nutritional information. Thirty-one companies hoped on board in the inaugural year, showcasing the Tick on 140 products. Over 25 years, a whopping 2,000-plus products spanning 80 food categories sported the logo, making it a household symbol Down Under. However, in 2015, the Tick program was phased out as nutritional labeling became standard on food items, alongside the advent of the new Health Star Rating System. Sadly, I see this as "same, same but different", as we say. This system doesn't get my naturopath tick.

The Pros and Cons of Butter

Pros: Butter is close to nature

Cons: Although butter has many health benefits, it is calorie-dense and is saturated fat.

The Pros and Cons of Margarine

Pros: I see no pros in margarine.

Cons: Think about this. Margarine production involves a complex process, starting with vegetable oils that are typically liquid at room temperature, such as soybean, sunflower, olive oil, palm oil, and so on. These oils undergo a series of steps, including hydrogenation, where unsaturated fats are converted into saturated fats by adding hydrogen atoms. They pump in hydrogen under heat and pressure to attach to where no hydrogen atoms are on the chain links. This process solidifies the oils, giving margarine its semi-solid consistency. Emulsifiers and flavourings are then added to enhance texture and taste. However, heating vegetable oils during hydrogenation and other processing stages can lead to the oxidation of the oils. This oxidative process can cause the formation of free radicals and breakdown products, leading to the oils becoming rancid, which is a fancy word for rotten. Rancidity alters the taste and smell of margarine and reduces its nutritional quality. To lessen this, manufacturers often use antioxidants and strict quality control measures to minimise the risk of rancidity and give better stability and shelf life. The thing is, they are so far from nature that it's scary. If you think the "olive oil" spread is healthier, sadly, they do the same process to get the liquid oil to solidify. These never get my naturopath tick.

What's the solution? You can make your own like I do.

My Butter Recipe

I make my butter. I buy an unsalted block of butter wrapped in paper and leave it out to soften. I leave it out to soften. I don't use a microwave, so if leaving it out isn't an option, we may want to warm it in a cool oven to soften it slightly.

Once it is soft, I put the block of butter into a container and then equal parts of olive oil. I don't measure it; I estimate. Then, I use a hand whisk to mix it. By blending the two, the olive oil mixes with the butter.

I then have a product that stays soft in the fridge and spreads easily. How much olive oil we use depends on how soft it is in the end; I find about equal parts oil and butter to be a good texture. By making our butter this way, the good Omega-6 and Omega-9 balance out the butter's saturated fats. I haven't heated the butter, so there are no trans-fats and better, yet it still tastes like butter!

GOOD SUGARS BAM

The average person eats more than fifty kilograms of sugar per year! Refined sugars are addictive and immunosuppressive and will destroy the ability of your to regulate blood sugar and insulin metabolism. Anything more than five kilograms of sucrose per year accelerates ageing, creates a breeding ground for yeast and fungus in the gastrointestinal tract and will leach important minerals from vital organ reserves. I'm not talking about natural sugars in fruits and vegetables. I'm talking about the crappy refined sugars.

Refined sugars are hidden in everything – packaged and processed foods are particularly dangerous because, in most cases, we aren't even aware of the sugars we're eating. Sadly, good plant sugars like monk fruit and stevia are being bastardised and misrepresented today. Take monk fruit for stevia or instance. Erythritol (Ah-REETH-ra-tall) is created when yeast ferments glucose from corn or wheat starch. Read our packets; sadly, most commercial monk fruit and stevia products contain around 1% of the actual fruit, and the remaining 99% is erythritol from corn. Yes, it is corn, not monk fruit or stevia. Eat close to nature, and our body knows how to handle the "real" sugars.

Stevia

Stevia is widely considered safe when used as a sweetener. It is about 300 times sweeter than sugar and has no calories. It comes from the "sweet leaf" plant, so some consider it a "natural" rather than an artificial sweetener.

Aspartame and sucralose, by contrast, are cooked up in a lab. The stevia plant is part of the Asteraceae family, related to the daisy called sweet leaf, which is native to New Mexico, Arizona, Texas, Paraguay and Brazil, where people have used leaves from the stevia bush to sweeten food for hundreds of years. While we can think, yay, natural, it isn't natural if we're buying a blend that's

99.8% Erythritol, a fermented sweetener made from genetically modified corn, with a pinch of refined stevioside powder.

Yes, stevia can be processed, mixed with chemicals, blended in a hundred ways and still legally be called "stevia". So be careful and read the labels.

Xylitol

Xylitol doesn't spike blood sugar or insulin, and it's said to starve the plaque-producing bacteria in our mouth and feed friendly microbes in our digestive system. Xylitol stops bacteria from living by starving it, and acids are not created, which alters the pH. Xylitol is a naturally occurring alcohol in most plant material, including many fruits and vegetables. It is extracted from birch wood to make medicine. It's also widely used as a sugar substitute in "sugar-free" chewing gums, mints, and other candies. So, again, we think, yay!

However, while xylitol is widely used, sorbitol is the sweetener most commonly used in sugarless gums because it is cheaper than xylitol and easier to make into commercial products.

Sorbitol

So, what is sorbitol? Sorbitol is a naturally occurring sweetener synthetically extracted from glucose. It's a laxative, drawing water into the large intestine and stimulating bowel movements. The not-so-sweet outcomes can be flatulence, bloating, cramping, and other abdominal discomforts.

I won't touch any sugar-free products. They will never get my naturopath's tick. Get the body working right and eat close to nature.

Coconut Sugar

Coconut sugar has a lower glycaemic index (35) than white sugar (60 to 65), and it doesn't spike our blood glucose, and insulin-like table sugar does. Honey and agave syrup are low on the glycemic index scale too.

Coconut sugar contains healthy fats that are known to help prevent high cholesterol and heart disease. Inulin is a type of dietary fibre that helps keep our gut healthy, prevent colon cancer, and balance our blood sugar. While standard table sugar is pure sucrose, coconut sugar only contains about 75% sucrose. Coconut sugar is a good option.

Maple Syrup

Maple syrup is a less harmful version of sugar, like coconut sugar. Its basic ingredient is the sap from the sugar maple or various other species of maple trees.

It consists primarily of sucrose and water, with small amounts of the monosaccharides glucose and fructose from the inverted sugar created in the boiling process. Maple syrup is about as sweet as sugar. It also has the same antioxidant and anti-inflammatory properties as green tea, which is also a superfood. Maple syrup offers great health benefits, just like blueberries, red wine, and tea. It's still sugar, though, so use it in moderation.

Agave

Agave syrup is a trendy new sugar and much higher in fructose than plain sugar, and it has a greater potential to cause adverse health effects, such as increased belly fat and fatty liver disease. It contains 60 calories per tablespoon – versus 48 for table sugar – but we can use less of it because it is about 1.5 times sweeter than sugar. Nutritionally, agave syrup is like high-fructose corn syrup. So, agave is not so cool.

So, what's the best solution to sweeten?

Stevia is the healthiest option, provided it is solely from the sweet leaf plant. Natural sugars like maple syrup, coconut sugar, molasses, and honey are also less harmful than regular sugar as they are closer to nature, and the body knows how to deal with them.

Is there more to nutrition? Absolutely. But this is the BAM to get us and keep us on track.

> *Eat sugars that are close to nature, and the body knows how to deal with them.*

DIGESTIVE ENZYMES BAM

Digestive enzymes play a critical role in breaking down food into nutrients that can be absorbed and utilised by our body. Produced primarily in the pancreas, stomach, and small intestine, these enzymes help the digestion of carbohydrates, proteins, and fats into smaller molecules that can be easily absorbed through the intestinal lining. Food particles can remain undigested without enough digestive enzymes, leading to discomfort, bloating, and nutrient deficiencies.

> **The best sources of digestive enzymes are often found mainly in fruits.**

The best sources of digestive enzymes are often found mainly in fruits. Raw fruits like kiwifruit, pineapple and paw paw are rich in natural enzymes that aid in their own digestion and can also support the digestion of other foods consumed alongside them. Pawpaw (papaya) and pineapple contain proteolytic enzymes such as papain and bromelain, which help break down proteins and promote overall digestive function. Green kiwifruit is an absolute favourite of mine as it contains an enzyme called actinidin, like the enzyme found in pineapples known for breaking down proteins.

Kiwifruit is my favourite food source of enzymes because once pineapple, papaya, or kiwifruit are cut, their enzymes, such as bromelain in pineapple and papaya and actinidin in kiwifruit, remain effective for a limited time. A kiwifruit is the perfect size to cut and eat in its entirety, whereas if we cut a pineapple and store some, we will miss out on the enzymes in the stored portion. We will still get the other nutrients but not the much-needed enzymes.

While we are on kiwifruit, eat the skin. The skin of kiwifruit is rich in dietary fibre, which promotes digestive health by helping with regular bowel movements and may help lower cholesterol levels. The skin contains great amounts of vitamin C, an antioxidant that boosts immune function, supports collagen production, and aids in the iron absorption. Vitamin E, another antioxidant in kiwi skin, helps protect cells from oxidative damage and supports overall immune function. Kiwi skin also contains folate and antioxidants like polyphenols.

Why care about polyphenols? These antioxidants protect cells from oxidative damage caused by free radicals, reducing inflammation and lowering the risk of chronic diseases such as heart disease, cancer, and neurodegenerative disorders. They also help relieve symptoms of inflammatory conditions such as arthritis and inflammatory bowel disease. Polyphenols also support cardiovascular health by improving blood flow, reducing blood pressure, and lowering LDL cholesterol levels. They may also promote healthy ageing by protecting against age-related cognitive decline and supporting overall brain health. Yes, I am a big fan of kiwifruit.

GUT MICROBIOME BAM

The gut microbiome is found everywhere, inside and outside, and it's like a protective mechanism. The gut microbiome refers to the diverse community of microorganisms, including bacteria, viruses, fungi, and protozoa, that inhabit the gastrointestinal tract. This complex ecosystem plays a crucial role in our body processes, including digestion, nutrient absorption, metabolism, and immune function.

The gut and brain communicate through a complex system called the gut-brain axis. This connection happens through nervous, immune, and endocrine pathways. The gut microbiome, comprised of various bacteria in our digestive system, produces substances that affect brain function and behaviour.

This communication happens through the vagus nerve, which links the gut and brain. The gut microbiome can activate this nerve, sending signals that impact mood, thinking, and actions. The gut bacteria produce neurotransmitters like serotonin and dopamine, which are our happy hormones.

Psychiatry Professor Ted Dinan coined the term psychobiotic in 2013. It explores using probiotics and prebiotics to improve mental health by targeting the gut-brain axis. Yes, restoring our gut chemistry and healthy gut microbiome may be possible to improve our brain function and emotional wellbeing.

> **Restoring our gut chemistry and healthy gut microbiome may be possible to improve our brain function and emotional wellbeing.**

The gut microbiome also affects the immune system, producing molecules that can affect brain function. Imbalances in the gut microbiome have been linked to conditions like depression, anxiety, and Alzheimer's disease.

We know that the gut influences so many body systems, yet people don't realise that we have prebiotics, probiotics, and postbiotics. There has been great promotion of probiotics for many years now, and people who get bloated and crampy or gassy, belly fat, constipation, and diarrhoea tend to think, OK, I need some probiotics. So, they buy probiotics from the local health food shop. But they don't realise they still need to eat the right foods. Prebiotics feed the probiotics so that they can flourish and then produce the postbiotics. Focusing on eating the following foods can help get our gut balanced and working for us instead of against us.

Prebiotics

Foods with healthy amounts of fibre, such as beans, whole grains, and certain vegetables, break down in our body to create substances that help probiotics to grow and thrive within our gut. All plants contain fibre, but not all fibre is prebiotic.

To be classified as a prebiotic, the fibre must pass through the GI tract undigested and stimulate the growth and activity of certain 'good' bacteria (the probiotics) in the large intestine.

What are the best soluble fibre foods that help?

- Dandelion greens.
- Jerusalem artichokes.
- Garlic.
- Leeks.
- Onions
- Psyllium husks
- Beetroot
- Asparagus
- Legumes
- Barley
- Whole oats
- Apples contain pectin, which is a soluble fibre
- Burdock root
- Flaxseeds
- Wheat bran
- Seaweed
- Sprouts
- Blueberries
- Green kiwifruit (skin on)

Since the fibre content of these foods may be altered during cooking, try to consume them lightly steamed or raw to gain the full health benefits. A combination of both raw and cooked, even nibbling on some of the raw while the rest is cooking, is a simple solution.

The goal is to eat 30 different plant foods daily to diversify our gut microbiome. Sadly, most people are not having even 30 different plant foods a week.

> **The goal is to eat 30 different plant foods daily to diversify our gut microbiome.**

It's time to count them up. Eating tomato sauce (ketchup) does not count as eating tomatoes (and yes, some people think that way). We need plant foods to feed our microbiome.

If we look at the healthiest populations on the planet in modern times, they're in the five blue zones (watch it on Netflix), and all five blue zones are 90 per cent plant-based.

I love travelling to Asia, where the plant is the centrepiece and the meat is the sideshow. Take a breath if you're a meat lover. Imagine just starting to eat 2-3 plant-based meals a week. You can go cold turkey, provided your head is around it. I promise your body will appreciate the change.

Why do we need to understand it? What we restrict, we crave. Set ourselves up for long-term success, and integrate slowly!

So, we have the prebiotics, which are the fibre. These are also the pungent foods. Garlic, leeks, onions, ginger, and cayenne chilli are also excellent prebiotics.

Probiotics

Probiotics are living microorganisms found in certain fermented foods, such as yoghurt, sauerkraut, kimchi, tempeh, and miso which are crucial to good digestion. Our digestive tract and overall wellness depend on a healthy balance of good bacteria and other microorganisms in our gut microbiome. We have about 100 trillion tiny critters living in our intestines.

> *Supplement with a Tribiotic, not a Probiotic.*

Postbiotics

Postbiotics are the waste left behind after our body digests prebiotics and probiotics. Healthy postbiotics include nutrients such as vitamins B and K, amino acids, and substances called antimicrobial peptides that help to slow down the growth of harmful bacteria. Other postbiotics are short-chain fatty acids to help the good bacteria flourish.

One last note on good bacteria: Alcohol damages it and causes dysbiosis (the balance of good and bad bacteria). I'm not saying no to alcohol; instead, think about how your body works and that drinking after work could be knocking out your gut microbiome and not helping your mental health and capacity to deal with the daily stresses of life.

> *What we restrict, we crave.*

ASSIMILATING AND ELIMINATING BAM

The end goal of good food is to assimilate and eliminate efficiently. When the body struggles with assimilating and eliminating properly, it can lead to a range of health challenges. Poor assimilation, or the body's inability to absorb nutrients effectively from food, can result in nutritional deficiencies, weakened immune system, and reduced energy levels. Poor elimination, such as constipation or sluggish bowels, can lead to toxin build-up in the body, causing bloating, digestive discomfort, and overall feelings of sluggishness.

> **Poor assimilation... can result in nutritional deficiencies, weakened immune system, and reduced energy levels.**

Let's talk poo. Yes, it's a naturopath's favourite topic. Why? It is one of the easiest ways to see what's happening in the body. I remember when I first graduated, I was doing a consultation on a patient who had a bad case of psoriasis. I was looking at his skin and checking his irises (which we use to help diagnose through iridology), and I asked, "Do you poo regularly?" He said yes. I looked at his skin and irises and thought, no, you don't. So, I asked how often do you poo? He said every Thursday. In his mind, he was regular. He was a meat eater, and that's fine, but he was in trouble eating two to three meals a day and not eliminating. From that patient on, I changed the way I asked that question to "how many times a day do you poo".

How many times should we poo a day? Think about an animal or a baby. They eat, and then they poo. When we chew and swallow our food, it heads towards our stomach. The ileocecal valve down at the gateway from our small to large intestine is triggered to open. What is in our small intestine moves into the large intestine, and what is in the large intestine moves toward the rectum, ready for elimination. If we eat two to three meals daily, we should eliminate two to three times daily.

If toxins don't come out through our pee and poo, it comes out of our skin. Poor assimilation and elimination can contribute to weight gain, skin issues, and an increased risk of chronic diseases. Everything in this chapter has been to help us assimilate and eliminate effectively so that our body can perform at its peak.

> *It's not what we eat that matters. What matters is what we digest, assimilate and eliminate.*

INTERMITTENT FASTING BAM

Let's talk about intermittent fasting. It is a naturopathic principle to have a fast day a week. Today, intermittent fasting has become a fad. It's a good fad; however, some scary variations are showing up.

Intermittent fasting involves cycling between periods of eating and fasting. Several methods are available, including the 16/8 method, the 5:2 diet, and alternate-day fasting. When coupled with herbs to support detoxifying body systems, intermittent fasting can be effective, and it gets my naturopath tick.

One of the key benefits of intermittent fasting is its ability to promote weight wellness and metabolic health. By restricting the time food is eaten, intermittent fasting can help regulate insulin levels, improve insulin sensitivity, and promote fat burning. Intermittent fasting has also been shown to support cardiovascular health by lowering blood pressure, improving lipid profiles, and reducing inflammation. It can improve cognitive function and brain health. As well as to support longevity and cellular health by activating autophagy, the process that removes damaged or dysfunctional components and promotes cellular renewal. I'm all about ageing well. This is why I do 'nutritionally supported' intermittent fasting.

> **I'm all about ageing well. This is why I do 'nutritionally supported' intermittent fasting.**

Like everything, when it becomes a fad, it gets bastardised. There are different versions of it, and people do things that aren't necessarily naturally balanced. A study by The University of Toronto found that the ever-popular 16/8 and 14/10 can increase binge eating.

Naturopaths traditionally recommend a fast day a week, a rest day, where we rest our digestive system. The difference is that we prescribe herbs when we recommend a fast day. We prescribe herbs to help support our detoxifying body systems and adrenal glands.

Why do we do a fast day with herbs? The bottom line is that we want to stay in the alkaline corridor, which I discussed earlier in the book. The alkaline corridor is when we eat alkaline-forming foods and are close to nature most of the time while managing our life stresses in ways that we can stay within the boundaries. The body works for us instead of against us. Helping to reduce inflammation, support detoxification, and improve cellular function, ultimately supporting great health and vitality.

With the stresses of life, we are kicked in and out of the alkaline corridor all day, every day. What we care about as naturopaths is how fast you return to it once you're kicked out. That's what matters.

When we're in the alkaline corridor, everything works properly. When we're out of it, our bodies are under stress, cortisol spikes, and we get out of balance. So, we want to do everything to keep us inside the alkaline corridor. If we don't eat, we stress our body. Stressing the body spikes cortisol, and people trying to lose weight by intermittent fasting could be causing more of a problem. Cortisol is the stress hormone that overrides everything. When intermittent fasting is done correctly, it is supported by adaptogens and herbs that help to detoxify our body systems

Imagine we have a body that's out of balance through stress, worry, overwork, hormones, and so on. We eat less, exercise more, and make a smaller body with a higher percentage of out-of-balance. The body then goes, I have to protect myself from this, and it does it by increasing visceral fat. So, we can have somebody smaller but still with a higher body fat percentage than someone bigger.

So, what's the answer? Intermittent fasting is great—I'm a big fan—but it just needs to be done properly. By the way, we can't detox our body. All we can do is support our body's natural detoxifying system. Supported fasting gets my naturopath tick, but stressing the body through calorie deprivation does not.

To intermittently fast, I support the body's natural detoxifying body systems with adaptogen herbs.

Adaptogens are special plants that help our bodies handle stress and stay balanced. They've been used forever in traditional medicines like Ayurveda and Traditional Chinese Medicine. These plants work by helping our bodies deal with different kinds of stress, whether physical, emotional, or from the environment. Adaptogens can help keep our cortisol levels in check, boost energy, and improve overall wellbeing. Some popular adaptogenic herbs include eleuthero, ashwagandha, rhodiola, holy basil, and Siberian ginseng, ashwagandha. An important note is that naturopaths never prescribe adaptogens singularly. We always prescribe them in a synergistic blend. As I write this, there is a rise in people using herbs like ashwagandha singularly, and it's frustrating because they will not get the results they are expecting.

Some of my favourite herbs to support the detoxifying body systems include dandelion, milk thistle, burdock root, ginger, and turmeric. Dandelion is known for its diuretic properties, helping to flush toxins from the kidneys and liver. Milk thistle contains a compound called silymarin, which supports liver health and helps to regenerate liver cells. Burdock root is rich in antioxidants and helps to cleanse the blood and lymphatic system. Burdock root helps to clean our skin from the inside out. Ginger is valued for its anti-inflammatory and digestive properties, aiding detoxification by promoting healthy digestion and elimination. Turmeric, with its active compound curcumin, supports liver function and has powerful anti-inflammatory and antioxidant effects, making it beneficial for overall detoxification and immune health. The inner leaf of the aloe vera plant contains polysaccharides, helping with digestive support.

When it comes to herbs, I use complete plants, like turmeric, not just isolated curcumin on its own. Mother nature gives us herbs in balance. All the constituents are there for a reason. When we try to isolate a particular component like the pharmacy industry likes to do, we move away from nature, and that's why we get complications, where using the whole plant generally doesn't. Mother nature is the clever one, and I trust her.

Supported fasting gets my naturopath tick. Stressing the body through calorie deprivation does not.

I understand if you've tried intermittent fasting before and found it challenging. It can be. So, let the moon help you fast, especially if you're a perimenopausal or post-menopausal woman. It could be that we're not running with the moon cycles. What do I mean? Our body runs a blood cycle, a biological cycle, and a moon cycle. Fasting three weeks out of the month will be easier for us than one week in a month. Let me explain.

> **Let the moon help you fast, especially if you're a perimenopausal or post-menopausal woman.**

Intermittent fasting aligned with the moon's cycles offers an easy way to wellness, particularly for peri or menopausal women. With the moon's cycle mirroring our 28-day cycle, syncing intermittent fasting with moon phases can enhance our results. If you no longer get a period, try planning intermittent fasting in line with the moon's cycles.

The New Moon begins of the fasting cycle, aligning with the first day of menstruation. During this phase, the body naturally focuses on cleansing and detoxification, making it an ideal time to initiate intermittent fasting.

As the moon moves to its first quarter, known as the Waning Moon, the body enters a phase of heightened detoxification and weight loss potential. This period, characterised by the gradual reduction of the moon's lit surface, corresponds to the body's natural preference to eliminate excess substances accumulated over the weeks before. Aligning our fasting with this lunar phase may allow us to experience better weight loss results and metabolic benefits.

The Full Moon, representing the peak of the lunar cycle, signals the body's elimination phase. This period, lasting approximately three days, is crucial for detoxification and weight loss. During the Full Moon, fasting can support the body's natural processes of elimination, helping to remove toxins and metabolic waste.

As the moon moves to its third quarter Waxing phase, fasting should cease, and the focus should shift to the assimilation phase. This phase is all about nourishment and replenishment, encouraging us to eat whole, nutrient-rich foods to support great health and well-being. By aligning our intermittent fasting with the moon's cycles, peri- or menopausal women can improve results by tapping into the natural rhythms of the moon's cycle to support detoxification, weight management, and overall vitality.

> *Use the moon to help you intermittent fast, especially if peri or post-menopausal.*

WEIGHT LOSS AND MUSCLE GAIN BAM

Weight loss is often simplified to a straightforward equation: calories in versus calories out. While this principle forms the basis of managing body weight, the reality is far more complex. Beyond simple maths, the body's hormonal balance, particularly stress hormones, shapes how we gain, lose, or maintain weight.

Psychological, emotional, or physical stress, triggers the release of hormones like cortisol. This hormone, the body's main stress hormone, plays a significant role in metabolism and fat storage. When stress becomes chronic or prolonged, cortisol levels can remain high, leading to physiological responses that influence our weight.

High levels of cortisol encourage the storage of visceral fat, particularly around the abdomen, which is associated with increased risks of metabolic disorders such as insulin resistance, type 2 diabetes, and cardiovascular disease. Cortisol can interfere with appetite regulation, often leading to cravings for sugary or high-fat foods, further complicating weight management.

Balancing stress hormones is crucial in achieving sustainable weight loss. This involves not only managing stress levels through mindfulness, meditation, using adaptogen herbs, and getting adequate sleep but also addressing the underlying causes of stress in our lives. Regular mindful movement, discussed later in this book, can also help regulate cortisol levels and promote overall wellbeing.

The quality and composition of our diet plays a pivotal role in hormonal balance and weight regulation. Diets close to nature, rich in whole foods, fibre, lean proteins, and good fats, support stable blood sugar levels and promote satiety, which can help lessen cortisol spikes and regulate appetite. On the other hand, diets high in refined sugars, processed foods, and crappy fats can exacerbate hormonal imbalances and contribute to weight gain. Aim for balanced health, eating close to nature 80% of the time.

> **Beyond diet and exercise, adequate rest and recovery are essential for hormonal balance and weight management.**

Beyond diet and exercise, adequate rest and recovery are essential for hormonal balance and weight management. Sleep deprivation, for instance, disrupts the body's hormonal regulation, increasing cortisol levels and impairing metabolic function. Prioritising consistent and restorative sleep patterns supports overall health and helps our body manage stress effectively. We know how good we feel after a good night's sleep and how well we function the next day. That's why Good Rest is our next focus.

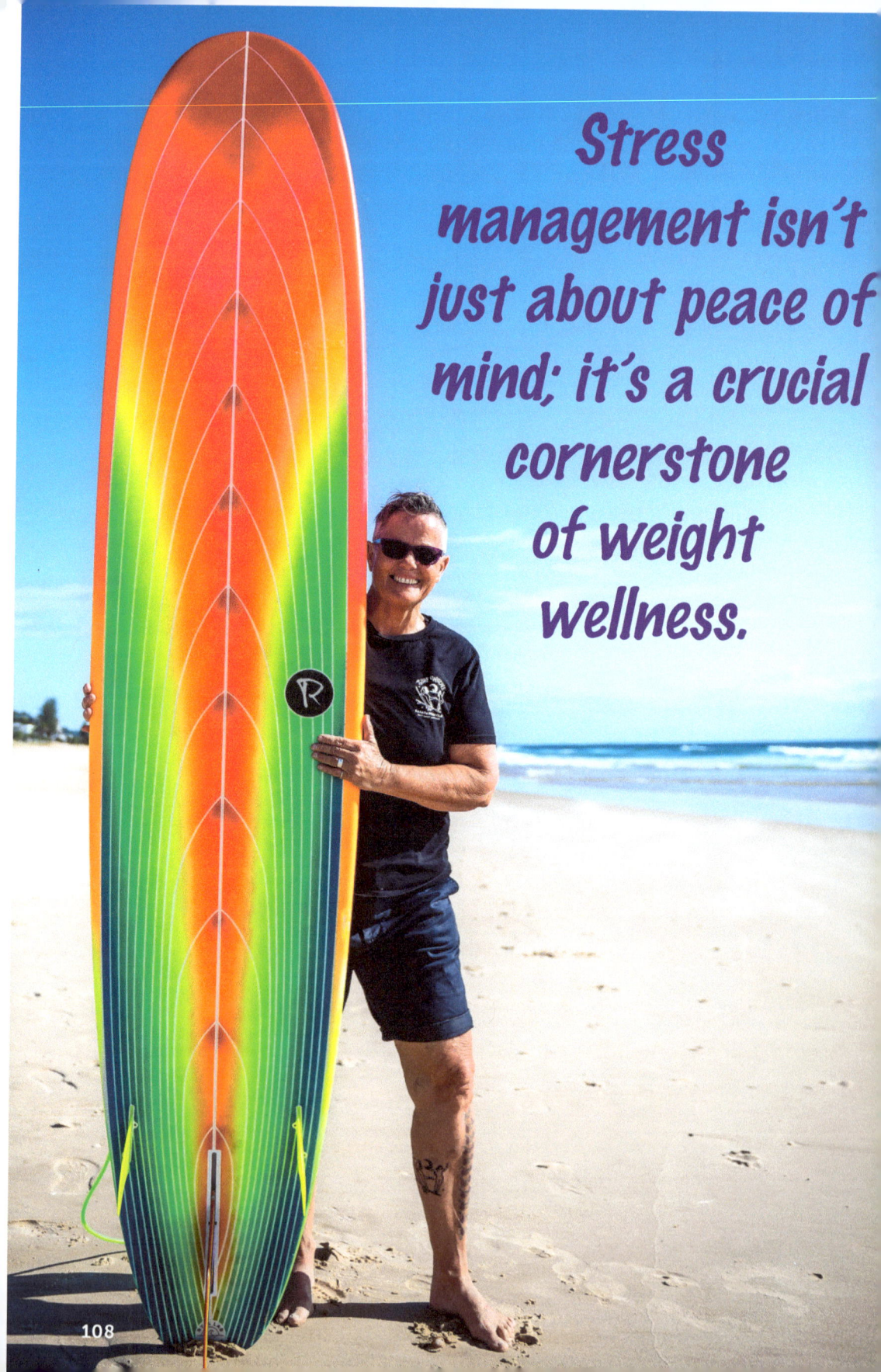

GOOD REST BAM

Good sleep is crucial for our health. When we sleep well, our bodies can repair themselves, boost our immune system, and keep our hormones balanced. Sleep also helps our brains work better, improving memory, focus, and decision-making. It reduces stress and makes us feel happier, lowering the chance of anxiety and depression.

Sleep is also crucial for brain health and preventing dementia. Plus, it's essential for physical performance and recovery, whether playing sports or just going about our day. Without enough good sleep, we might feel tired, grumpy, and less productive, and we could be at risk for health problems like obesity, diabetes, and heart disease.

Prioritising sleep is not negatable. The number one change I made in my life after burning out was to respect my sleep. All my friends know that I take sleep seriously and that six nights a week, I will happily play hard and leave early to get the sleep I need.

> **Prioritising our sleep is not negatable. The number one change I brought to my life after burning out was to respect my sleep.**

Key factors in achieving great sleep are a healthy sleep environment, maintaining consistent sleep habits, managing stress, and addressing any underlying health issues.

Our body has a circadian rhythm, the internal clock that regulates sleep-wake cycles. It follows a roughly 24-hour cycle that responds to light as a signal to be awake and dark as a signal to fall asleep.

I always get ten before 10. What's ten before 10? Dr Andrew Huberman suggests starting the day with 10 minutes of morning sunlight to regulate the circadian rhythm every day. I have the ritual of heading straight to the surf when I wake for a sunrise surf. It helps set my circadian rhythm plus gives my mental health a boost to take on the day.

To strengthen the circadian rhythm even more, Huberman suggests spending an additional 10 to 15 minutes in the late afternoon or early evening sunlight.

Avoiding bright light two hours before bedtime and creating an utterly dark sleeping space can also make it easier to fall asleep. When our eyes sense light, even a little bit, they signal to our brain to stay awake and stop producing melatonin, a hormone that helps us sleep. So, sleeping in a dark room helps our body make more melatonin, which means deeper and better sleep. Also, too much light at night messes up our body's natural rhythm, making it harder to fall asleep and stay asleep. By keeping our sleeping area dark, we can improve how well we sleep, making us feel happier, think better, and be healthier overall.

Balancing stress hormones and getting great sleep is the most important thing we will do all day.

Want more energy... get better sleep.

Want to lose weight... get better sleep.

Want to age slower... get better sleep.

Want to be less stressed... get better sleep.

Stress directly impacts all body systems. When we're stressed, and our adrenal glands don't get a chance to recharge correctly, it can affect our gut chemistry, mental health, energy, and sleep. It just keeps going.

Cortisol is the new buzzword. It's a hormone made by the adrenal glands. Cortisol receives so much attention because more and more people are burning the candles at both ends, and their adrenals are paying the price.

Cortisol in our body helps to maintain everything from our blood pressure to our immune function and anti-inflammatory processes. The amount of cortisol released is regulated and dependent on how our body handles stress and determines how we wake in the morning.

At night, our cortisol levels drop. As morning nears, they rise, peaking soon after we wake. This surge helps release stored energy, like glucose, to fuel our day. Cortisol jumpstarts our metabolism, giving us the energy to tackle the day. But if cortisol stays high due to stress, it can disrupt this cycle, causing us to drag our butt in the morning.

> **When we experience chronic stress, an overproduction of cortisol occurs. As a result, we overtax our bodies, which shows in our sleep. The stress loop continues.**

Producing cortisol is a good thing, and it's part of our survival mechanism built into our fight-and-flight ability. The challenge is that our bodies feel constantly attacked when we burn the candle at both ends. Lots of constant little stresses are beating us. When we experience chronic stress, an overproduction of cortisol occurs. As a result, we overtax our bodies, which shows in our sleep. The stress loop continues.

One result of the overproduction of cortisol in our bodies can be the inability to handle or recover from stress. Blood sugar levels drive energy levels, moods are all over the place, blood pressure can rise, weight gain or loss can occur, the immune system can be overtaxed, and we end up living in survival mode.

At some point, we need to bring our bodies back to a place where they can regenerate. I know we will not slow down anytime soon; I won't, anyway. So, we need to support our bodies while we maintain the pace at which we are going. In a perfect world, we'll realise that this pace can't be maintained without taxing our bodies unless we think and act in prevention. In my experience, people don't change until they hit burnout or some nasty illness manifests to wake them up. That's what happened to me, and today, I do what I write about in this book to stay balanced and live from a place of prevention.

Some of the common factors that increase the production of cortisol are sleep deprivation, overuse of caffeine, improper nutrition, constant stress, and simply burning the candle at both ends.

Supporting our adrenal glands and controlling our cortisol levels can be as simple as learning to relax by having regular massages with essential oils or taking a nutritional and herbal tonic to recharge as we go. Overproducing cortisol makes us feel hungry and can lead us to crave foods that feed the problem.

> **Controlling our cortisol levels can be as simple as learning to relax by having regular massages with essential oils or taking a nutritional and herbal tonic.**

In the clinic, the class of herbs that we work with is called adaptogens. I touched on them earlier. An adaptogen is an herb that helps our body, and particularly our adrenal glands, adapt to the stress it is experiencing. So, if we are experiencing high blood pressure, adaptogens help to normalise our blood pressure. The same goes for lifestyle ailments like blood sugar imbalances and so on. We cannot make stress magically go away, but we can support our bodies to manage the stress and help our bodies function more normally.

One of the primary adaptogen herbs that I have used in the clinic is Siberian Ginseng. It is one of my favourites. You may have heard of Ginseng in the past, but the Korean Ginseng is generally a lot more energising than the Siberian Ginseng. If we come from a place where we are adrenally tired, Korean Ginseng can be too stimulating and bring us right up, and then we can crash down the other side. This doesn't happen with Siberian Ginseng. It is a great adaptogen that helps to tonify our body. It increases energy but at a sustainable level, which is important. It's all about looking long-term and regenerating our body to a place where it can handle all that life throws at it. It's not just looking for a quick fix.

Remember, naturopaths never prescribe adaptogens singularly; we prescribe them in synergy. We are not one body system. We are a body of body systems. Treat the body holistically and gain the maximum benefits by bringing it back into balance.

> **Treat the body holistically and gain the maximum benefits by bringing it back into balance.**

In ayurvedic medicine, they talk of the "'destroyer of weakness", the adaptogen herb Shilajit. Nepali Shilajit is a thick, viscous material that oozes from the cliffs of the Himalayas. It's rich in many phytochemical nutrients and contains the miracle molecule called dibenzo-alpha-pyrone. Sounds impressive, and it's very cool. It is particularly efficient at transporting nutrients into the body and helping mobilise heavy metals and expel them out of the body. Combine Nepali Shilajit with other Ayurvedic adaptogens such as Ashwagandha (Indian Ginseng) and Amla, and we have a rejuvenating blend of herbs that helps to tonify body systems and bring us back to excellent health.

Liquorice root, recognised for centuries in traditional medicine systems like Traditional Chinese Medicine (TCM) and Ayurveda, is celebrated for its adaptogenic properties. As an adaptogen, liquorice root helps the body adapt to physical, emotional, or environmental stressors, thereby supporting overall resilience and wellbeing. It contains compounds such as glycyrrhizin and flavonoids that contribute to its therapeutic effects, including anti-inflammatory, antioxidant, and immune-modulating properties. Liquorice root is commonly used to support adrenal health, balance cortisol levels, and promote gut health by soothing inflammation and protecting mucous membranes. However, it is essential to use liquorice root cautiously and under guidance due to its potential for side effects, particularly when taken in large quantities or for extended periods, as it's high in potassium.

In Russia, Rhododendron is another great adaptogen that scientists have extensively researched for use with athletes. Extreme exercise can be taxing on all body systems, and elite athletes are especially interested in improving their body systems' function so that they can perform better.

Schizandra is also an extremely powerful adaptogen. Each one of these adaptogens has different characteristics of phytochemical nutrients, sometimes over 50 different ones, that perform different functions and have nutritional benefits and effects on many different organs in the body.

Tribulus is also a herb used extensively with athletes under stress to help with energy levels and increase strength and performance. Tribulus can also be found in formulas designed to help increase libido because of its ability to help regulate blood flow. One of the first things that leave us when we are stressed is our libido. It's like our bodies say, "Look, I am already running tired, and the last thing I have energy for is having more kids in my life, so the desire for sex can disappear. Our adrenal glands also produce our boy and girl hormones. Burn the candle at both ends and see how quickly your libido disappears. If your libido is already gone, start with a good adaptogen tonic.

> **Burn the candle at both ends and see how quickly your libido disappears.**

Magnesium is the first mineral we burn up when we stress out. Black strap molasses is the unrefined form of molasses, and it contains more nutrients than molasses itself. It is closer to nature and has an extremely rich mineral and trace mineral profile. Minerals in our body function as coenzymes, helping to ensure proper vitamin utilisation. So many daily ailments can be traced back to a mineral deficiency.

Nobel Laureate Dr Linus Pauling said, "One could trace every sickness, every disease, and every ailment to a mineral deficiency!" I absolutely agree.

> I am a big fan of taking adaptogens at bedtime because I want to allow my body to enter that adrenal-recharging sleep.

I am a big fan of taking adaptogens at bedtime because I want to allow my body to enter that adrenal-recharging sleep. If we use adaptogens during the daytime, they'll adapt to what we're doing. If we use them when we're busy in the morning, for instance, they will help keep us energised and focused. Take them at bedtime, and they'll help keep you grounded for better restorative sleep. The trick is to take them right as we are lying down for sleep as they adapt to what we are doing. If we go to bed to read or do other fun things, wait to take the herbs as we are ready to sleep.

Our adrenal glands need between seven and nine hours of sleep a night to recharge properly. Naturopathically, we say that if we were doing broken sleep between 2am and 4am, we know that cortisol is out of balance. Sleeping through the night is the goal. If you stir or your cat walks over your head like my HarLee does at night, we should be able to go back to sleep quickly. If we lay there wide awake, that's not good.

Ideally, we are in bed and asleep by 10pm. I know the night owls are thinking, but I like to stay up late. Well, feel free to keep doing that. I used to do that, too. I used to say we sleep when we're dead. But studying to be a naturopath and working with clients this way for over three decades, I know that if we don't get enough sleep, we get off this planet earlier.

What happens then is we wake up in the morning after a night of broken sleep? We're not refreshed because our cortisol has been out of balance, and our bodies haven't been able to replenish effectively, so we drag our butt out of bed. Our energy is low for the day, we don't deal with stress properly, and we stay in that loop.

If we're having trouble getting to sleep, we're likely low in calcium. That's why a glass of warm milk before bed can help. Other good sources of calcium include dairy products (such as milk, cheese, and yoghurt), leafy greens (such as kale and spinach), fortified plant-based milks, and certain fish (such as sardines and salmon) and seeds. Sesame seeds are an excellent source of calcium, and there's more usable calcium in a teaspoon of sesame seeds than in a glass of milk. Put them on a salad of the day and in cooking. They are great for us if we do or don't have broken sleep.

If we're having trouble staying asleep, we've gone past the calcium stage and are now generally low in magnesium. Magnesium is the first mineral that we burn up when we stress out. Magnesium-rich foods include nuts and seeds (such as almonds, blackstrap molasses, and pumpkin seeds), legumes, whole grains, leafy greens, dark chocolate, and some fish. It is a water-soluble nutrient, so it's dumped easily with cooking.

> **If we're having trouble getting to sleep, we're likely low in calcium… If we're having trouble staying asleep, we're generally low in magnesium.**

If you're into aromatherapy, you'll want to use more calming essential oils to take the edge off your nervous system so you can switch off. Essential oils like lavender have been shown in studies to help balance out cortisol while we're sleeping. So, any essential oil blends containing oils like lavender are going to be beneficial for getting to sleep. I created my Serenity Blend, a serene combination of Frankincense, Geranium, Lavender, and Ylang-Ylang essential oils, to assist in creating a calm environment conducive to setting up well for sleep.

If you're having trouble staying asleep, we've gone past the flowery essential oils and need more heavy wooden root and wood oils, such as sandalwoods, cedar woods, and vetiver. Vetiver is my favourite essential oil. It grounds a busy brain. It's not a sedative. It just allows our body or brain to ground so we can think of one thing at once: sleep. My Sanity Saver blend includes Vetiver, Patchouli, Ylang Ylang, Geranium, and Australian Sandalwood, and it has been created to stop our minds from racing so we can focus. It helps to restore some peace and balance to our lives during the busiest and most stressful times. Perfect to use at bedtime, during the day, or in the workplace to still a busy mind.

> **If you're experiencing broken sleep...cortisol is probably out of balance. Stress and broken sleep don't allow our bodies to recharge properly.**

My Sanity Saver blend is the one I designed for my constitutionally "go fast" ADHD brain. To stay grounded and productive, switch off, and sleep to recharge appropriately at night is a blessing. If you're experiencing broken sleep and it's been going on for a while, cortisol is probably out of balance. Stress and broken sleep don't allow our bodies to recharge properly. Check out the Resources page at the back of this book for links to my other books and aromatherapy blends.

ADAPTOGENS ARE NATURE'S RESILIENCE IN A BOTTLE.

While on the topic of ADHD... I am a 'go fast person'. My mind races, and I am spontaneous, fun and creative. I'm always doing a dozen things at once, and the pace with which I like to get things done makes most people's heads spin—and I have no intention of slowing down anytime soon! I see my ADHD as my superpower.

There has been a marked increase in the diagnosed cases of ADHD over the last few years. Recognition of ADHD symptoms and their impact on daily functioning has resulted in healthcare professionals being more likely to identify and diagnose ADHD in people who may have been overlooked in the past.

The diagnostic criteria for ADHD have evolved over time, leading to a broader understanding of "Go Fasts" and its presentation across different age groups and genders.

Whether we have a "go fast" mind diagnosed or not, managing that pace is essential. I've been through burnout, and now I know that to keep up the pace, I need to support my adrenals in advance.

> **Whether we have a "go fast" mind diagnosed or not, managing that pace is essential.**

Vetiver is known for its grounding effects; it is beneficial for mental exhaustion and helps to relax a scattered mind. It benefits the workaholics and the "go fasts" like me. I use it with Jasmine, Bergamot, Sandalwood and Geranium, which I call my 'Sanity Saver' blend. I use it in my office in a room vaporiser, and before I go to sleep, I rub a few drops diluted with body oil into the soles of my feet for a good night's rest. It's not a sedative; it grounds us to focus on one thing at a time and settle down to finish what we are working on without trying to do ten things at once and not achieving anything other than driving our stress levels through the roof. It's about focusing and recharging. It helps stop our mind from racing to get a good night's sleep.

Some of the same oils in my Sanity Saver blend were used in a three-year study with children with ADD/ADHD. The 2001 study by Dr. Terry Friedmann highlighted some great results using aromatherapy essential oils. Whenever the kids felt 'scattered', they inhaled the oils, and it was found that this settled the brainwaves back into regular patterns and improved their academic performance and behaviour. The results were as follows: Lavender increased performance by 53%, Cedarwood increased performance by 83%, and Vetiver increased performance by 100%. (If you're particularly interested in using essential oils with kids, my book Calm Kids explains how they work and how to use them.)

Many adults have similar habits to some of these 'go fast' kids: They have a lot going on, their attention is scattered in many directions, and they try to do a dozen things at once. I've found that these same oils are particularly effective at helping anyone drop their stress levels and focus. Grounding ourselves with my Sanity Saver Blend is the place to start.

A quick word on alcohol. Having a wine or beer in the evening to wind down disrupts sleep patterns, affecting the quality and duration of rest. Relying on alcohol to unwind after a challenging day can be counterproductive. While alcohol may initially induce feelings of relaxation, it ultimately interferes with our brain's ability to enter deeper, more restorative sleep stages.

The power move is not to wait; come from a place of prevention. Use adaptogens, aromatherapy, and nutrition to set yourself up for great sleep. It is my highest priority of the day. It's that important.

Being a Grounded Go Fast is my Superpower!

GOOD PLAY BAM

As I already shared, in the 1980s, I pushed myself too hard in the corporate world, neglecting my health and values. I kept going until a car accident forced me to stop and rethink my life. I remember my mum saying, "Jen, what are you doing?" I thought I was all good. See, I had all the 'stuff' that says I'm successful: the right job, house, car.

Today, I see many people making the same mistakes I did, so focused on success that they ignore their wellbeing. Would you hire someone like that?

Instead of brushing off concerns about overworking, we should listen to our friends and family. They might see something we don't.

> **Instead of brushing off concerns about overworking, we should listen to our friends and family. They might see something we don't.**

Remember when we dreamed of being in the very situation that causes us stress today? Or did we dream of something different and wonder how we got here? There was a time when we all felt like life would be an incredible adventure. What happened to that excitement along the way? Our adrenal glands need us to lighten up.

In his book Anatomy of an Illness, Norman Cousins shares how he used laughter to overcome a crippling disease that doctors thought was incurable. Cousins, a writer, diplomat, and editor, was diagnosed with ankylosing spondylitis in 1964. Doctors told him there was no known cure, and stress might have caused it. Remembering a book he read about how negative emotions could harm the body, he wondered if positive emotions like love, hope, and laughter could help. Cousins left the hospital and started a program focused on enjoying life and positive emotions. It worked, and he lived another sixteen years. His story shows the importance of attitude and enjoyment in health.

Stress is recognised for its ability to raise blood sugar levels, posing risks for people with diabetes. Today, Type 2 diabetes continues to rise As of 2017-2018, it was estimated that around 25% of Australian adults aged 18 years and over had either diagnosed or undiagnosed prediabetes, according to data from the Australian Bureau of Statistics (ABS) and the Australian Diabetes, Obesity and Lifestyle Study (AusDiab). This suggests that approximately 1 in 4 adults in Australia may have prediabetes .In this condition, blood sugar levels are higher than normal but not yet high enough to be classified as Type 2 diabetes.

In 2003, a study examining the impact of laughter on blood sugar levels revealed promising findings for those with Type 2 diabetes. Researchers observed that increased laughter may help the body's ability to process sugars from food. The study involved 19 diabetics and five non-diabetics whose blood sugar levels were measured before and after eating an identical meal. Participants then attended a comedy show or a monotonous lecture on separate days. Post-meal blood sugar levels were lower after the comedy show and higher after the lecture, indicating that laughter effectively reduced blood sugar levels for both groups.

It's important to consider our environment during mealtimes. Many people habitually eat dinner while watching the evening news, which mainly carries doom-and-gloom stories. Eating meals and taking in that negativity can impact physiological processes. If we choose to watch or listen to something during meals, opt for a light-hearted or funny show to encourage healthier blood sugar levels. When I sit for lunch each day, I'll watch a comedy. I'm serious about taking in the funny side of life.

> **I'm serious about taking in the funny side of life.**

If you're into aromatherapy, we can bring some life into our workplace and help everyone better manage daily pressures and frustrations by using essential oils in a room vaporiser. I designed my 'Play More' blend for when we are taking life or ourselves too seriously. It is the perfect blend for lightening up and enjoying life again, to regain the feeling that we are living and not just existing. It is ideal for the boring, burned-out perfectionist. It contains Sweet Orange, Geranium, May Chang and Grapefruit essential oils. Geranium oil has been found to actively calm the glucocorticoids, after which the adrenals send other chemicals, which flood the brain with serotonin and cause people to calm down. The oils won't impact our ability to behave and respond professionally and competently, they'll just take the edge off the anxiety, which ultimately helps everyone to think more clearly and respond even more effectively

> "If we are in a bad mood, go for a walk.
>
> If we are still in a bad mood go for another walk."
>
> — **HIPPOCRATES**

MINDFUL MOVEMENT BAM

The truth is I am no exercise queen or expert. I do, however, move my body mindfully every day. I know that it helps me feel good mentally and emotionally. Exercise boosts self-esteem, improves our mood, helps us handle stress better, and helps us age better.

Being 63, as I write this, I'm more focused on moving daily. In the past, I had periods where I could not be bothered. A big part of that came from my inner rebel saying no. When I was in the army, every time we screwed up, we were punished. The punishment was exercise-based with push-ups, burpees or running. Exercise, to me, was punishment. I needed to reframe it for my health.

MINDFUL MOVEMENT BAM

If our body is adrenally tired, the last thing we want to do is to flog it. Going for a 10K run or working it hard at the gym with a heavyweight session won't help restore the adrenal glands. Your adrenal glands are restored with mindful movement. Movement from things like Tai Chi, Qi Gong, Yoga and walking instead of running. We need to replenish the adrenals if we're running that tired. So mindful movement isn't necessarily hitting the gym like our brain thinks it should have in the past.

Mindful movement also needs to be fun. When I was 56, I took up surfing. I found such joy in surfing. I get to do a full-body workout every session—cardio and full-body weight training. If you want a visual, taking off on a wave is like doing a push-up downhill about 20km per hour or faster on a totally unstable surface. To surfers, that part is worth standing up on the board, riding the wave at one with nature and fully present in the moment It is pure bliss and fun. We cannot have another thought in our head when we are surfing. I found my peace in surfing, and I found a way to move my body daily that I enjoyed.

Here's the tricky part: when life gets busy and stressful, exercise is the first thing we tend to skip. If it's not enjoyable, we'll miss it. Have you ever had a morning where the plan was to work out, but your mind was racing with tasks, leaving no time or energy for exercise? Or you promised yourself you would hit the gym after work, only to feel too tired when the time came. It's a common cycle.

> *"We can't stop the waves, but we can learn to surf"*
>
> JON KABAT-ZINN

When our energy is sluggish, we need to move our bodies. However, we need to move in a way that replenishes the adrenals, not drains them more. If tired, we need to spend we energy to gain energy.

> **If tired, we need to spend we energy to gain energy.**

Apart from looking after our adrenal glands, we all know regular movement is crucial for staying healthy as we age. It keeps our muscles strong, joints flexible, and bones healthy, which helps prevent falls and injuries. Exercise also helps our heart and blood vessels stay healthy, lowering the risk of heart disease, stroke, and high blood pressure. Plus, it supports our brain health, reducing the risk of Alzheimer's disease and other types of dementia. I wrote earlier about studies showing the need to eat enough protein to build and maintain lean muscle and to help pump blood to our brain. Staying active and maintaining lean muscle mass can help us remember things better and keep our minds sharp as we age. So, making exercise a regular part of our routine is important for staying strong and healthy as we grow older.

If you don't like exercise like me, my 'Move Your Butt' aromatherapy blend could greatly support you. This energising blend is designed to help us move our buts (our excuses) so we can move our butt. It's a synergistic blend of grapefruit, lemon, and fennel essential oils that helps us stop being delicate, start being optimistic, and stand in our power to achieve our goals in life.

My wife Alice is the opposite of me. She loves exercise. She surfs, does beach runs and gets plenty of other mindful movement every day. It is a way that she channels her stress.

Check out the link on my Resources page to visit my wife, Doctor Alice MacKinnon, The Stillness Ninjas website. She has a range of videos where we can do therapeutic movements like chair yoga at work or some Qi Gong moves. It is a simple movement that replenishes the adrenal glands.

> "If we could give every individual the right amount of nourishment and exercise, not too little and not too much, we would have found the safest way to health."

HIPPOCRATES

THE WINDOW OF WELLNESS

As I close out this book, one last thought is that comfort is killing us. It is hard to watch people selling themselves short and settling for a "good life" when they are living resigned and cynical. So many have lost the fight and given in over the last few years.

What stops us from having a great life is having a good life. But at any time, we can say enough, just like I did in my 20s and again in 2020. We can get uncomfortable and bring the change we want in our lives. If you see someone with the energy, vibe, health, and all the things and ways of being you want, take a stand, get uncomfortable, learn from them, and bring the learnings into your life. At least start and build on the little wins.

THE WINDOW OF WELLNESS

Please also understand that "the window of wellness" is always open. It's always the right time to take the first step to get back on track. Also, remember the sayings, "Off track, back on track" and "no story, no problem" I wrote about earlier in the book. Giving ourselves a hard time for being off track won't help. Acknowledge ourselves for taking the courage to come back on track.

> **Giving ourselves a hard time for being off track won't help. Acknowledge ourselves for taking the courage to come back on track.**

Will it be a big ask sometimes? Yes. Is it worth it? Absolutely. The secret is to start. We know that if we keep doing the same thing, we won't be in the same place in 12 months. There is natural attrition in nature. We'll be in a worse place in another 12 months, whether with health, finances, fitness, or anything else.

If you're thinking, I don't have time even to do the bare-arse minimum; you will pay for it with your health. Be it in advance now, coming from a place of prevention, or ultimately shortening your life. We always pay. I choose to pay now and enjoy great health in the future.

I also know that what we think about, we bring about. It may be time to change your thinking and make health a priority. We have the time to live in a place of prevention and not wait to get sick.

Some people reading this will get all excited, learning something new like this and think I will take all of this on 100% from the start. Please stop and take a breath. I want sustainable health and longevity for everyone, so make lifestyle changes that will stick versus trying to do it all at once. Stop and start kills our spirit. Little successes day in and day out will build consistency, and consistency is what brings the results, especially with our health. Is there more to it than this? Yes, but if we start with the BAM, 80% of our physical, emotional and mental health will begin to come back into line.

Celebrate all the wins, no matter how small. If we nail drinking our 3 litres of water today, go us. If we managed 2 litres when we generally have none, that's huge and needs to be acknowledged. We lose hope and give up if we don't feel we are making progress. Celebrate every win, no matter how small. Enjoy those dopamine hits and use them to stay on track.

Set health and wellbeing goals and tweak them as you go along. Set the weekly goals to a size that you can feel the little wins to keep you motivated. It is important to set ourselves up for success from the start. I want people to achieve long-term lifestyle changes rather than short-term fad attempts. Don't go for short term Band-Aids. Go for long term real sustainable change.

> **Don't go for short-term Band-Aids. Go for long-term real sustainable change.**

If you are truly ready for a full Reset, reach out to me and tell me why. If you are wondering if you are ready for a full reset, you are not ready yet, and that's OK. So go for the BAM. Start there.

Before burning out, I was an alcoholic, propping myself with anything I could grab to manage the stress in my life. I prided myself on working hard and playing harder. I was not a nice person and had no sense of peace. I was constantly trying to prove myself to others to get their approval. Burning out and that car accident ended up being the best thing to happen to me, and I doubt I would be alive today if I had not gotten that wake-up call. I didn't make 100% change overnight. I started and consistently built layer on layer, where today I feel bloody fantastic, and I am proud of my journey.

If you're reading this and thinking, I don't have the time, as Gandhi said, "I have so much to accomplish today that I must meditate for two hours instead of one." Success isn't convenient. There will never be the right time or enough time to start. It's a choice.

THE WINDOW OF WELLNESS

It's time to make ourselves the number one priority in our life. It's not selfish. Its self-respect.

I wish you to find peace and flow while sticking close to the mark 80% of the time. That is achievable and sustainable for even the busiest person.

For some extra support while breaking the stress loop, use my F*CK The Stress aromatherapy blend.

This blend embodies the vibe of my F*CK The Stress Book. This essential oil blend banishes self-doubt, and boldly declares "F*CK The Stress."

I Am Un-Messable!

It's my time!

It's a choice.

It's time to make ourselves the number one priority in our life.

It's not selfish. Its self-respect.

THE 7 STEPS TO SANITY CONDENSED

When I wrote my book, The *7 Steps to Sanity*, back in 2002, I wrote it as a prescription for modern living with the unique insight of someone who has not only travelled the road to burnout and back but has also as a health-care practitioner. It was designed to be an easy step-by-step lifestyle plan that was realistic, achievable, and easy to incorporate for everyone who feels the pressure of trying to balance the demands of work with the rest of their life.

With the *7 Steps to Sanity* complimenting the Bare Arse Minimum approach, I thought I would share a condensed version as a bonus to this book to provide you with further actionable and easy-to-remember steps to *F*CK The Stress*.

Stressed-Out or Burnt-Out?

Stress is one of those things that we all experience to different degrees and through various symptoms and ailments, which can make it challenging to diagnose and treat. Insomnia, anxiety, depression, hypertension, headaches, heart palpitations, diarrhoea, or constipation, loss of libido, aches and pains, exhaustion, behavioural issues, cognitive difficulties, anger, substance abuse, feeling disillusioned, withdrawn and helpless are just some of the manifestations of long-term stress.

Dr Edward Creagan, an oncologist at the Mayo Clinic, describes the response to prolonged stress as being 'like a football player who has repetitive trauma in the game. One hit, and he'll survive, but add up week after week of hits in a season, and he'll be hurting. He may not be able to handle it anymore.'

Our bodies give us clues to let us know when we are under too much negative stress, but we tend to be so busy and so focused on the external needs and demands of our lives that we don't have time or can no longer hear, what it's trying to tell us. The problem with our stress-related coping behaviours and physiological responses is that they tend to set off sequences of events that trap us in adverse health effects. Let me give a couple of common examples.

When stressed, we often reach for things that will give us short-term energy hits or comforts; stimulants such as coffee, alcohol, nicotine, sugar, or fatty foods are usually the first things we seek. The problem is that the things we reach for to relieve our stress cause more stress. When we are experiencing stress, it's because (among other things) our adrenal glands are tired, so we grab a coffee, cigarette, glass of wine or packet of chocolate biscuits to calm and comfort us, but as we devour these things, our body systems are further taxed by dealing with the toxins, fats or sugars, which further fatigues our adrenals and reduces our ability to cope. So, on we go. Fighting fires and causing more damage along the way until we get to the point where we can no longer get through the day without the stimulants we are now dependent on to help suppress the symptoms we are experiencing.

Think about the effects of stress on our blood pressure. When we are experiencing stress, our adrenal glands release the stress hormone cortisol, which mobilises excess fatty acids, metabolic wastes and glucose stored within our arteries. When our cortisol levels are too high for too long, the probability of atherosclerosis (clogging of our arteries) increases dramatically. It's a vicious cycle: the stress causes high blood pressure, which releases more cortisol, which in turn releases more toxins, which block arteries and increase blood pressure. We're living in the 'stress loop'.

Stress Overrides Everything

STEP 1 – RESPECT YOURSELF

Self-care is essential, yet often neglected as we prioritise the needs of others over our own. I call it the 'Burnt Chop Syndrome'. Why? Imagine cooking a meal of lamb chops and burning one. Who gets the burnt one on their dinner plate? If you're a woman reading this, it's probably you. The burnt chop syndrome sees us sacrificing our wellbeing to avoid disappointing others or due to feelings of unworthiness. Women tend to prioritise caring for others at their own expense. In our professional lives, this manifests as the 'I'll just finish this one thing' syndrome, leading to neglect of self-care. But there is a reason we're instructed to put on our oxygen mask first in an emergency on an aircraft. How can we look after others if we don't survive ourselves?

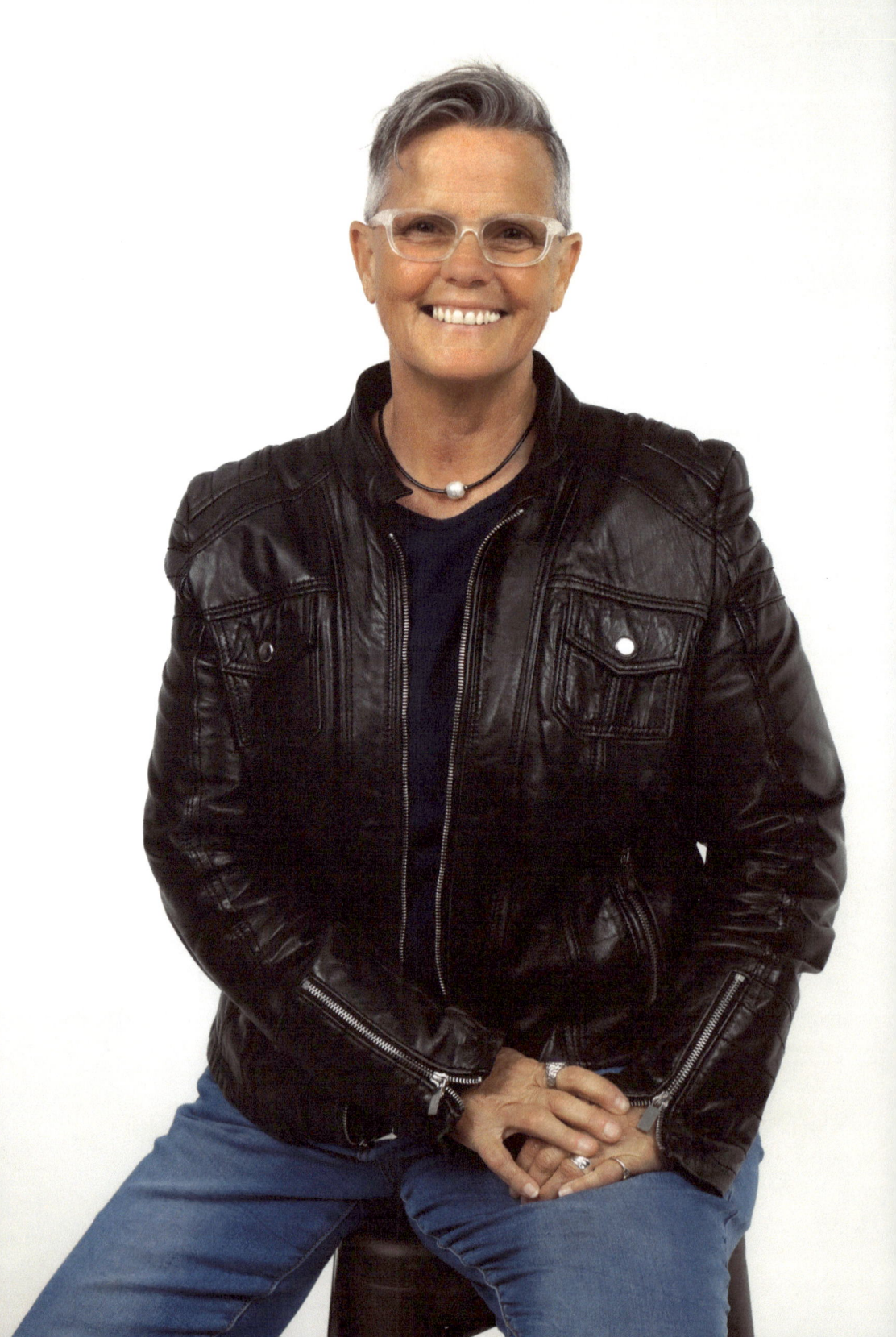

Learn to Say 'No'

Many of us struggle with saying 'yes' to every demand placed upon us; I sure did in the past. We believe that saying 'no' would brand us as selfish or inconsiderate. What if we respected ourselves enough to start saying 'no'? This doesn't suggest selfishness; instead, it shows an understanding of our limitations and a commitment to realistic expectations. It shows respect for our responsibilities and time constraints, showing ourselves and others that we prioritise integrity over overextension. It's a mature, responsible, and considerate approach; though admittedly easier said than done, it is worth learning and practising. If we choose to say no, own that no. If we decide to say yes, own the yes. Saying no and then guilt-tripping ourselves won't help in any way. Negative emotions like guilt are more damaging to our body than eating bad foods.

Ask for help

Facing truths can be uncomfortable but necessary. Many people find comfort in portraying themselves as victims of stress and overwork to gain sympathy. I, too, struggled with this, not wanting to appear weak. This reluctance led to more stress and then more health challenges. But now I understand that asking for help is a sign of wisdom, not weakness. It develops collaboration and empowers others, leading to more success and fun. Remember also that humans are service-orientated. We feel great when someone lets us help them. It's time for us to stop being selfish and let others help us. Reflecting on the toll not asking for help took on me, trying to be superhuman, today I've learned to park my ego, embrace vulnerability, and accept help.

I know that, at times, we get swamped at work with non-stop phone calls, social media and a flood of emails. It's like drowning in a sea of tasks. If we were drowning in the ocean, we would scream for help if we needed it. Why should drowning in life be any different? Choose to park your ego to the side and ask for help.

Growing up, I learned to be strong and independent to survive. This has been a great strength and a great weakness. It made it hard for me to ask for help when needed. Instead of admitting I was struggling, I'd say I was fine. But pretending only made things harder. Eventually, I got sick of struggling. I took a deep breath and asked for help. The response was amazing. I practised at the supermarket. When I go shopping, even if I know the location of the product I'm looking for, I find a staff member. I look them in the eye and politely ask if they can tell me where that product is. That began as a practice that is now a positive habit. Even asking for one thing on a shopping trip will be a great start. People are usually happy to lend a hand and feel they are of service when they do. Remember to thank them well for their help; you can make a difference in their day.

I should point out that asking for help differs from just dumping something on someone. Asking for help comes from our hearts, and they feel it. Dumping comes from the head. Before speaking, take a breath, get grounded, and feel the emotion. I know it's super easy to ask from the head. But when I don't ask from my heart, I generally get a no over a yes. Asking for help doesn't just benefit us; it gives others a chance to help, which feels good for them, too. Plus, teaming up with others can help us achieve more than we ever thought possible. So, don't hesitate to ask for help when needing a hand. You might be surprised by the support you get.

Asking for help is a sign of wisdom, not weakness

Words Work

Words hold immense power, shaping our experiences and wellbeing. Both internally and externally, our words influence our mood and attitude profoundly. Internal self-talk often leans towards self-criticism, impacting mental, emotional, and physical health. Redirecting this negativity involves first noticing and replacing harmful scripts with positive, affirming statements. How we speak to ourselves influences our experiences. Choosing positive words over negative ones shifts our focus and energy, transforming our mindset and approach to life. The secret is when we catch ourselves in a negative groove, think, "Awesome, I caught that one", and reframe it to the positive.

I remember in the 1990s reframing "no worries" or "not a problem" with "too easy". It was messy at first as I caught myself midsentence. Today, my default is that things are easy, not problems and worries.

When we catch ourselves, the secret is not to give ourselves a hard time, as that only reinforces the negativity. The more we catch and reframe, the faster we create a new default. The power move is to keep going, to let ourselves be "bad at it long enough to get good at it". That's how real change happens.

> *Every Master was once a Disaster... including me.*
>
> DAVID TS WOOD

Fear or Excitement

What slows our progress and prevents us from pursuing our dreams? For most people, it's fear of some kind. Fear and excitement evoke similar physiological responses; the distinction lies in our perception. The power move is to work with our breath and keep moving. How do we do that? We breathe. When we fear, we breathe shallow and fast; when excited, we draw in a deeper breath. Our body only knows what is going on by how we breathe. So, when I feel fearful and stressed, I draw in a deep breath and let myself feel really excited instead. Like Dory from Finding Nemo says, "Just keep swimming."

I live by the mantra, 'If it's hard to do, it's even more important to do it.' Despite appearances, even the most fearless people experience fear. They simply choose to keep moving and embrace "the excitement".

If it's hard to do, it's even more important to do it.

STEP 2 – FEED YOUR BODY

For many, food is a source of pleasure and indulgence, often leading to overeating. We eat for various reasons, a few of which prioritise providing our bodies with nourishing fuel. Many people's eating habits tend to be unconscious; we use food to fill emotional voids or help us fit in. Unfortunately, we often eat items we know aren't beneficial for our health, effectively using food to harm ourselves. It's strange that while half the world struggles to get enough food for survival, the other half grapples with an overabundance, resulting in obesity and related health issues. For more information, refer to the Good Food BAM earlier in this book.

Eating close to nature 80% of the time, keeps us in the Window of Wellness.

STEP 3 – MOVE YOUR BODY

A sedentary lifestyle can powerfully impact our physical and mental health. Physically, prolonged sitting and lack of regular physical movement contribute to weight gain, increased risk of obesity, and a higher likelihood of developing chronic conditions such as cardiovascular disease, diabetes, and musculoskeletal disorders. Muscles weaken, flexibility diminishes, and our metabolism slows down, further exacerbating health issues.

A sedentary lifestyle is associated with more stress, anxiety, and depression. Physical activity is crucial for maintaining a healthy weight and cardiovascular system and releasing endorphins that boost our mood and overall sense of wellbeing. Building in regular movement breaks, standing desks, and engaging in physical activities can significantly lessen the adverse effects of prolonged sitting and promote better physical and mental health outcomes.

How crazy is it that when we're busiest and most stressed, we neglect exercise, yet moving could help us channel stress and feel better?

Think about starting even a ten-minute lunchtime workout. Instead of eating at the desk, finding even ten minutes for physical activity is feasible. Many people work long hours without breaks, sacrificing exercise and relaxation. Bringing workouts into the workplace becomes crucial. Here are three simple exercises to give our body a lift and start to get us moving at work:

1. **Wall push-ups** are an effective upper-body exercise. Stand at arm's length from the wall, with arms shoulder-width apart. Maintain a straight posture, engage the core, and slowly lower ourselves into a push-up against the wall. Progress by bringing the hands closer together makes it more challenging.

2. **Air Squats** are ideal for toning our biggest muscles, the legs and buttocks. Stand facing the desk, with feet shoulder-width apart. Keep the back straight, push the hips back, and lower ourselves until our thighs are parallel to the ground—or as low as we can go. Return to the standing position. Focus on pushing the hips back while keeping the knees over the toes.

3. **Computer curls.** We can work our biceps at work using even a water bottle. Think about it—a 500ml water bottle is still half a kilogram and worth it. Sit upright or stand, with elbows tucking into our sides. Slowly raise the water bottle toward our shoulders, palms facing upward. Even low-weight, high-repetition movements can help build our muscles and ease computer-induced shoulder tension.

These workplace exercises seem trivial, yet they offer a boost in tone, strength, and energy. To maintain a consistent exercise regimen, it's crucial we find activities we enjoy. I love surfing for pleasure and exercise, and I do weights at home with a PT online. I'm not a gym girl, but I'll exercise to help my surfing. Never discount the value of incidental exercise. Every movement counts.

I need to also speak about 'skinny fat'. There is a difference between thin people, characterised by a low percentage of lean muscle mass and a high percentage of body fat, and those who are genuinely fit, boasting a strong physique with a high percentage of lean muscle and a low percentage of body fat. Despite appearing thin, people of this nature may have a higher body fat percentage, with them technically 'fatter' than people of a larger. This kind of fat is generally visceral fat.

I first learned about 'skinny fat' when I first burned out. I went to a health retreat to help my recovery, and on day one, we had a swag of health checks done on us. I remember a petite Asian woman who was there being so distressed because her results showed that she was grossly unhealthy and overweight. Where I was a larger and a more solid woman than her and came out with great numbers What I learned was that she was; skinny fat' and had a higher level of visceral fat from stress. This motivated me to start learning what was happening in our body with the effects of stress, which led me to study naturopathy. I had to understand what was going on.

Visceral fat, often referred to as 'hidden' fat, poses substantial health risks even in people who appear lean or skinny fat. This type of fat accumulates deep within the abdomen, surrounding vital organs like the liver, pancreas, and intestines. Despite not being visibly evident, unnecessary visceral fat increases the risk of serious health problems such as insulin resistance, Type 2 diabetes, heart disease, and certain cancers. Skinny fat people have a high proportion of fat relative to muscle mass and may have high visceral fat levels due to stress, sedentary lifestyles or poor dietary habits. Regular exercise, particularly resistance training, managing stress and a balanced diet are crucial in reducing visceral fat and improving overall metabolic health in skinny fat people. Go for muscular, fit and healthy, not skinny.

> *Never discount the value of incidental exercise. Every movement counts.*

STEP 4 - PLAY MORE

People have become way too boring and serious. Modern life often feels mundane, drowning out our childhood dreams and ambitions. Despite our initial enthusiasm for trying new things, we often find ourselves trapped in draining routines.

We are the leading cause of our energy loss. Ignoring our own needs, like eating well, exercising, and having fun, drains our vitality. Anything or anyone that makes us unhappy is an 'energy sucker', while things that make us feel good are 'energy givers'. We can notice what's draining our energy and replace it with things that help us feel alive and happy. Energy suckers can be anything from food to people or habits that don't energise us.

When it comes to people, we are said to be the sum of the five people we spend the most time with. We reflect the company we keep, influenced by the attitudes, behaviours, and energies of those closest to us. Surrounding ourselves with upbeat, fun, positive people can profoundly impact our outlook on life and personal growth. Positive people tend to ooze optimism, resilience, and a positive approach to challenges, inspiring us to nurture similar qualities within ourselves. Their encouragement and support creates a safe space for personal development and growth. We can become a force for positivity, helping to feed each other's happiness and success in meaningful ways. A great question to ask ourselves is, who do we hang out with most of the time? Are they energy givers or energy suckers? How do I feel before and after I spend time with the five people closest to me? It's worth asking that question regularly.

Life is full of challenges that can feel far from being fun. Waiting for the perfect moment to play and be happy is pointless because it might never come. We often think we'll be happier after reaching certain goals like marriage, career success, or travel. However, putting off happiness for the future is risky. There's never a perfect time. Instead, we can appreciate what we have now and choose to be happy in the present moment.

Playing more isn't just fun —it's a power move for great health!

STEP 5 – GET A LIFE

Our adrenal glands are taxed by all the physical and emotional stress that we experience. In Traditional Chinese Medicine, the adrenals are said to be where our Qi (life energy) lives, and when we run out of Qi, we die. So, the phrase 'get a life' has a very literal meaning.

As a naturopath, I see the adrenal glands as the main body system contributing to burnout. Throughout my years as a naturopath, more than 85% of the patients I treated showed signs of adrenal fatigue or exhaustion. Prolonged adrenal stress has been linked to headaches, backaches, insomnia, anger, cramps, high blood pressure, chronic fatigue syndrome and lowered immune system functioning resulting in re-occurring bacterial or viral infections. For women, prolonged stress is a major factor in thyroid and hormonal imbalances resulting in menstrual irregularities, menopause challenges, PMS, fibroids, endometriosis and fertility problems, and loss of libido is common in both women and men. The first thing to go when stressed is our libido. Our body says we don't have the energy to make a baby, so let's just shut that function down. Keep the stress up for long enough, and stress can also lead to the development of almost all disease states, including cancer and heart disease.

So, what are our adrenal glands? The adrenal glands are small triangular organs that sit like caps on top of each kidney, and they work like a bank account – we spend a little adrenal energy each day, and each night, with good sleep, we build up our reserves again. But the reality is that many people spend more than they re-invest, which means that most people are experiencing adrenal tiredness a lot of the time. The combination of prolonged stress, poor sleep and diet, overuse of stimulants such as tea, coffee, alcohol, and long working hours without rest or play is what we naturopaths call adrenal fatigue. It generally presents as dark circles under the eyes, and crappy energy, moods, sleep, weight, a compromised immune system and not feeling great in general.

You've undoubtedly heard of adrenalin and generally understand it is produced when the body is under stress. Adrenalin speeds up our heart rate, increases blood pressure, quickens our breathing and diverts blood from our digestive system to our muscles so that we can stand and fight or get out of there This 'fight or flight' response was beneficial in days gone by, such as when we had to catch and kill our evening meals. Imagine being confronted by a wild creature and having to fight for your life or run for it; this is where the adrenals kick in to give us the high-level surge of mental alertness, physical strength, and stamina that will help us survive. But these situations, as stressful as they were, would be resolved quickly. The stress response would subside, and life would return to normal, allowing our adrenals to recharge. Today, people are fighting different types of battles daily, which feel just as stressful in the absence of real-life and death situations. Everything from the daily commute to stress and pressures at work, relationship issues, the kids demanding "mum", financial stress, performance anxiety and environmental pollutants can tax our adrenal glands, and the trouble is that we are not getting the chance to recharge.

The human body can only take so much stress. If the stress does not stop, if the energy produced is not released appropriately, the adrenal (and other hormone-producing) glands will become exhausted. Our quality of life largely depends on how well we look after our adrenals. If we want to live a fast life, we can, and the only way we can sustain it over the long term is to look after our bodies, or we will crash and burn out, like I did. Quality relaxation and downtime daily are among the most important things we can do to recharge our adrenals. It's their job to keep us charged and ready to go for it, but if they aren't properly fueled when the pressure is on, we'll have nothing left to call on.

In my experience, stress, worry and emotional overwork are more exhausting and damaging to the adrenal glands and general health than most external or physical factors. Humans are good at internalising our stress, wanting to look good, efficient, and capable, and showing our colleagues that we can handle whatever is thrown at us. No one likes to be seen as not being able to cope, so we get on with it by suppressing our emotions. Because the human body can adapt and handle stress for extended periods, people think that how they deal with life is normal. The sad thing is that it often takes something drastic, such as total burnout, an accident or a severe illness, to shock us into action, modify our lifestyle and behaviours and restore balance. This was my story, for sure.

There's no magic pill that we can take to replenish our adrenals, but as we've discussed, there are adaptogen herbs that support them. However, regular and consistently good food, rest, and play will recharge us the best.

As I said, the adrenals work like a bank account. It's about balance, and contrary to what some people think, self-care and balance is not for wimps. Without fully functioning adrenals, we won't be functioning at our best and able to achieve all we want. We must start looking after our adrenal health to thrive in life. The great thing about this is that I'm not saying that we must slow down or give up on any of the plans and dreams that we have in life. We can still do it all and have it all. Today, I still power through life, and I get to support and balance myself so that I don't kill myself along the way or, like so many people do shortly after retirement, drop dead when we arrive.

When we run out of Qi, we die.

Self-care isn't selfish —it's essential.

STEP 6 – DO IT NOW

We often waste energy worrying about unfinished tasks, big or small, like cleaning the garage or starting a weight loss journey. Waiting for the 'perfect time' is a mistake because it never comes. So, if there's something I want to do, I choose it and do it now—even one little part of it. I know that we generally only procrastinate on the things that we don't want to do. The things we want to do, we magically find the time to do them.

Procrastination is common, even with simple tasks like making a phone call. We put it off, convincing ourselves it can wait until tomorrow. Delaying it overnight means we have a crappy sleep, and it only brings stress and exhaustion. When we finally act, we wonder why we waited so long as it generally goes better than expected. We wasted time instead of getting it done and feeling free.

Overwhelm often creeps in when we find ourselves standing still, frozen amongst the madness of tasks and responsibilities. It signals that we've stopped too long, allowing the pressures and uncertainties to build up. Yet, overwhelm carries a hidden message: it urges us to take that first step, however small, and to keep moving forward. Action is its antidote. Embracing overwhelm as a prompt for progress, we can recognise the power of every little step. No matter how small, each stride disrupts stagnation and moves us forward. Overwhelm then becomes a catalyst for growth, not a barrier, reminding us that in motion, we find our way through the challenges that once seemed overwhelming.

How do we get moving? We take a breath, wiggle our toes to get grounded, and take the first step. Don't wait for the perfect moment. Take that breath and just take one step and then another. If I had waited to have big blocks of time to go surfing when I was travelling the world nine months a year, I would never have gone. All steps forward count, no matter how small.

Many people feel overwhelmed and stressed at times, leading to physical symptoms like headaches and digestive issues. I call this 'chucking a 'poor me'. Our perspective on life plays a significant role in this cycle. By taking control of our emotions and outlook, we can become calmer, happier, and more flourishing.

Frustration from not adapting to changes can lead to anger and negative emotions. What creates frustration? Having expectations. A huge lesson for me to learn has been that my expectations are my expectations. I can never control everything or everyone, so why get frustrated when something doesn't go my way? Letting go of expectations, especially about situations or people, can lead to an easier life. While it's natural to have expectations, letting them control us keeps us trapped. All we can ever control is our response to what is happening. Expectations not met lead to frustration, anger, and ill health.

We can choose how we see things and let go of beliefs that hold us back. When frustration arises, try using essential oils. Realise that the world will not end if everything doesn't get done today. I designed my Chill Out blend, which contains Orange, Lime, and Ylang Ylang, to help us stay focused on the future but still remember to live for today.

Action is the antidote. Overwhelm becomes an opportunity for growth, not a barrier.

Speaking Our Truth

We can procrastinate at work and in our personal lives because we are scared to speak honestly. We're afraid of being judged or to lose our jobs, so we don't speak our minds. We talk from our head vs speaking from our heart. When we speak from our heads, we say what we think they want to hear vs speaking from our hearts, we speak our truth. People feel the difference and being honest takes courage and builds better relationships. It saves energy spent overthinking and analysing conversations. Stop wasting time and speak honestly from the heart with yourself and others. It's much more rewarding.

> *When we speak from our heart we speak our truth.*

STEP 7 – REMEMBER YOU'RE HUMAN

Have you ever heard the saying, "We are not playing for sheep stations"? It's an Aussie term that means no one is going to die and the world will not end because of what is happening right now. It means there is no need to be so intense about it, as the outcome is not worth risking everything for. It's our way of saying, "Let's not make a big deal out of this".

I was flying to Sydney for a speaking gig twenty years ago when all flights were suddenly cancelled. This caused mixed emotions because I was flying to Sydney to speak at a conference. With it out of my control, I knew I could not get there, and instead of getting upset, I accepted the situation and dealt with it as it unfolded. While standing in line trying to get another flight, I called the client, worked out a plan to help them in the future, and just dealt with it. I realised that stressing wouldn't change anything. Despite the setback and standing in line at the airport for a few hours, I connected with some epic women who are still precious friends today. The super cool thing is that I eventually closed a business deal with them, to design the signature scent for a hotel of one of the biggest luxury brands in the world. That deal would not have happened if not for that cancelled flight and if not handling how it all unfolded. All we can ever do is control our response to life and trust it, as it's always perfect; we just don't always know why it's perfect at the time.

From big challenges to small ones, how we view things and keep moving forward is up to us.

Work stress is a big issue, with Monday mornings being tough for many. People would rather die than go to work. Most heart attacks tend to occur early in the week, with Monday mornings being particularly high-risk. Research shows that the increased stress and anxiety of going to work after the weekend may contribute to the higher incidence of heart attacks during this time. As the weekend draws to a close, thoughts of returning to work, meetings, and responsibilities can bring feelings of stress, anxiety, and fatigue. Things such as Sunday sleep-in's, more alcohol and extra eating over the weekend, and the dread of going to work on a Monday make this a scary statistic. Mondayitis is more than just a passing feeling of reluctance; it can drastically impact our productivity, motivation, and mental health. The stress and anxiety related to returning to work after the weekend can lead to less job satisfaction, higher absenteeism, increased levels of burnout and can kill us. Chilling out and realising we are not playing for sheep stations is essential on every level.

I spoke with an executive who had everything that showed he was successful—the big house, holiday home, flashy car, and so on. But he wasn't happy. He realised he was working so hard to pay for everything he wanted that it kept him trapped. Having too much stuff complicated his life and didn't bring joy.

In Australia, homes, cars, and everything else are getting bigger even though families are smaller. People chase wealth and status, thinking it'll make them happy, but it often leads to stress and financial problems. Before buying more stuff, think about whether it will genuinely make you happy. What makes us happy is a sense of purpose and connection, not the stuff we accumulate.

> *Don't settle for quick-fix band-aids with health. There is no short cut. Work the root cause.*

THE 7 STEPS TO SANITY

Step 1. Respect Yourself

Step 2. Feed Your Body

Step 3. Move Your Body

Step 4. Play More

Step 5. Get A Life

Step 6. Do It Now

Step 7. Remember You're Human

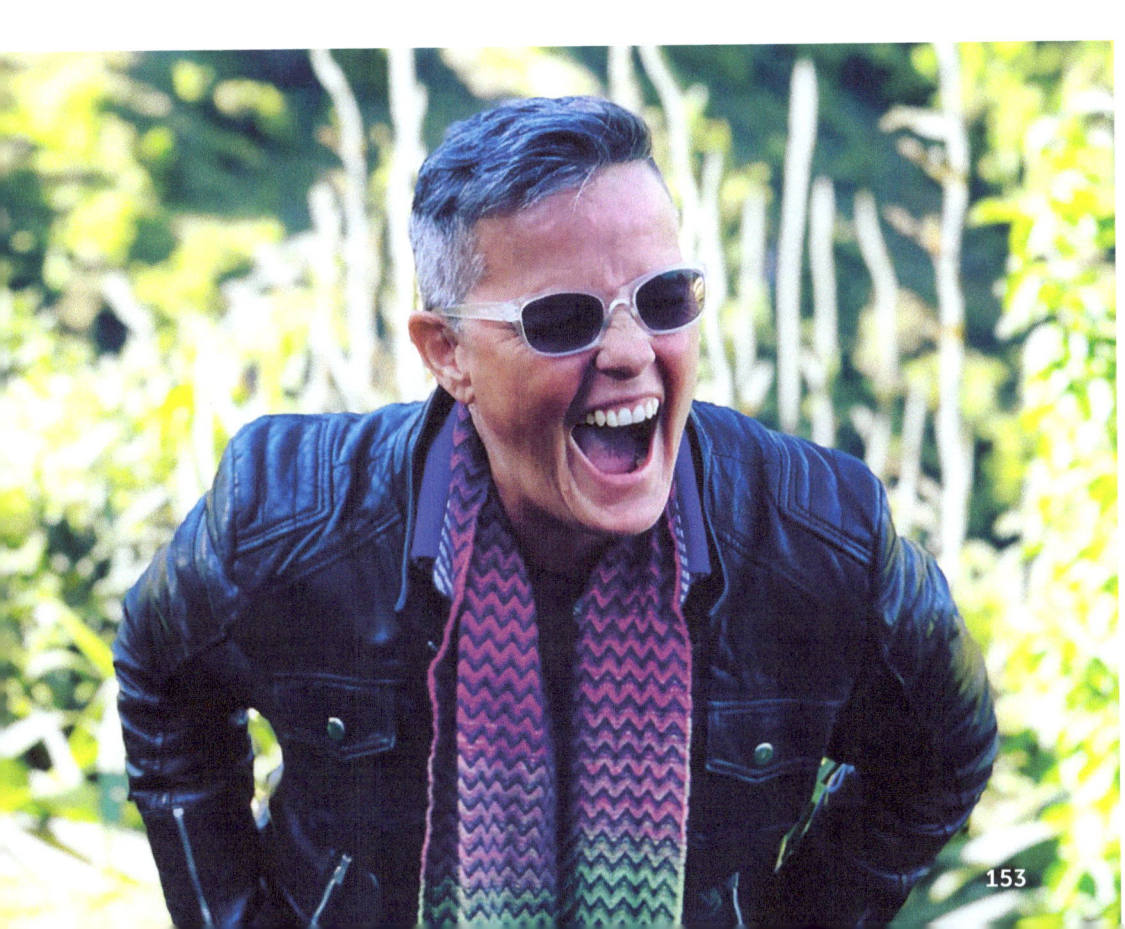

RESOURCES

Jen's Books

jenniferjefferies.com/store-books

- Amazing Scents
- The Aromatherapy Insight Cards
- Calm Kids
- The Scentual Way to Success

Jen's Essential Oils

jenniferjefferies.com/store-essential-oils

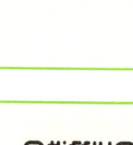

- F*CK The Stress Blend
- Sanity At Work Kit
- Sanity Saver Blend
- Chill Out Blend
- Play More Blend

Jen's Signature Range

- Live It Blend
- Love It Blend
- Get On With It Blend

Calm Kids Kit

- Breathe Blend
- Study Blend
- Calm Kids Blend

Jen's Habitat Kit

- Energise Blend
- Seduce Blend
- Serenity Blend
- Move Your But Blend
- The Surfing Unicorn Blend
- AVAB Blend

Jen's Coaching Programs

jenniferjefferies.com/inner-circle

RESOURCES

Jen's Online Programs
jenniferjefferies.com/store-online-programs

- Aromatherapy Insight Cards Course
- How To Boost Our Energy & Fire Up Our Life
- How To Sleep Our Way Out of Adrenal Fatigue
- Smart Sassy Seniors Live Recording

Jen's Podcasts
jenniferjefferies.com/podcast

- Healthy Life Hacks
- Smart Sassy Seniors

FREE eBooks By Jen
jenniferjefferies.com/freebies

- 7 Easy Protein Ball Recipes
- Healthy Life Hacks To Start thriving
- Healthy Life Hacks Podcast Show Notes: Episodes 1-200
- Pelvic Floor Prolapse Support

The 30 Day Reset Program
Jen recommends
jenjefferies.isagenix.com/en-au

Dr Alice MacKinnon Website
aliceionamackinnon.com

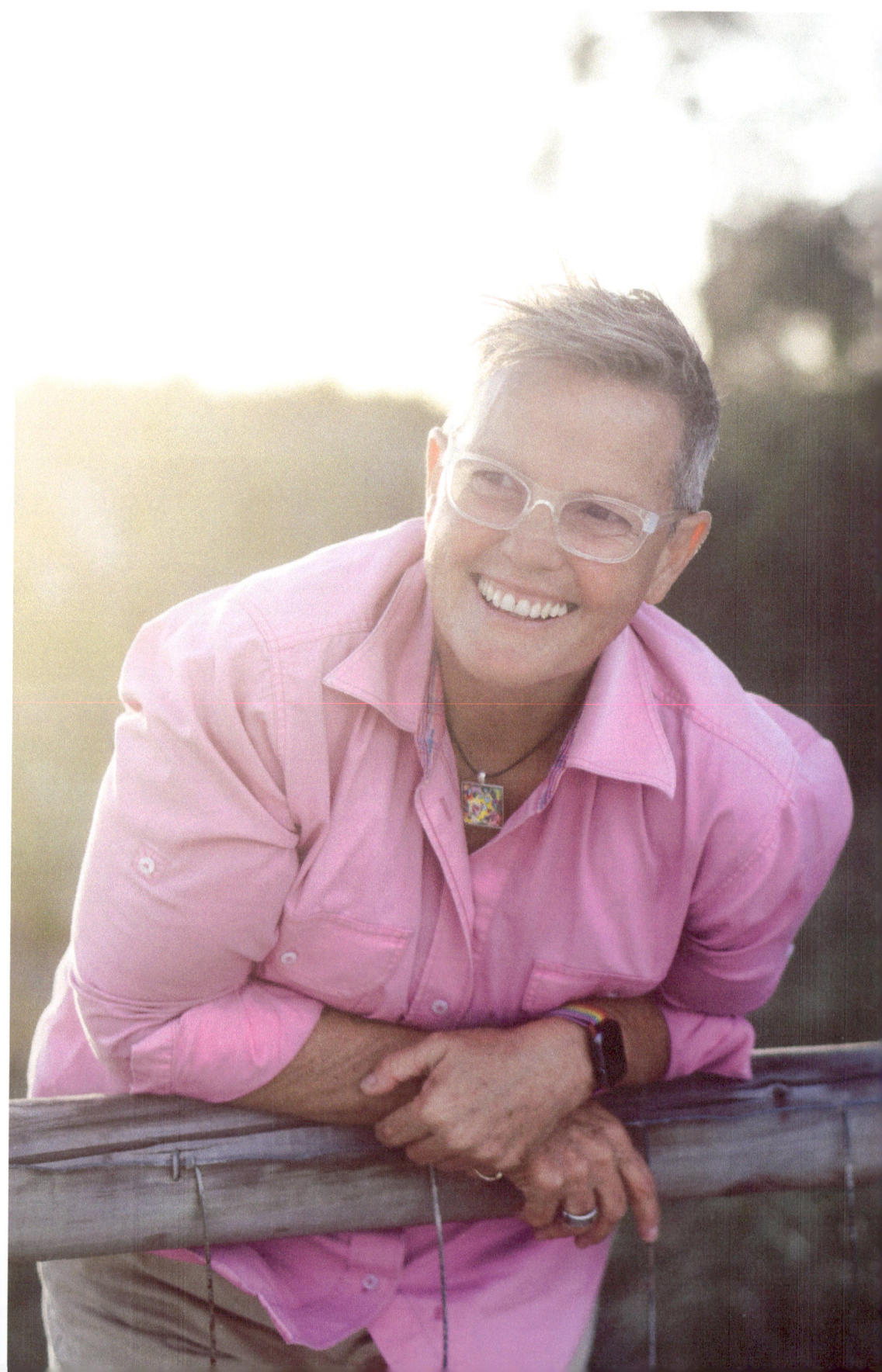

THANK YOU'S

To my wife Alice for always being my biggest support and for being such a bright light on this planet. Your courage to show up and fight the big fight to grow inspires me. I love you forever and always.

To my assistant and gorgeous friend Shane. You make my life easier, your steadiness amongst my "Go Fast" world helps keep me grounded. I love you dearly and I am so proud of you. My life is richer with you in it.

To my editor Amanda who nurtures the words and wisdoms of this kid who failed high school English, to be readable by you all. Your patience and help are treasured.

To Ingrid my book designer, I feel your heart in all that you do. That is a gift to this world.

My Digital Queen Anne, I am forever blessed to have met you and to have you on my team. You are a bloody gem and gorgeous soul.

To all of you who are in the game, showing up and putting your arse on the line to help others. Your courage inspires me, especially in a time when we become easy targets for those who have no skin in the game, and choose to try and hold us back. Remember to always shine brightly and never tone down your vibe for anyone.

About the Author

JENNIFER JEFFERIES

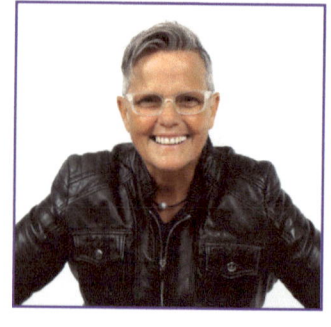

Jennifer Jefferies is The Present-Day Wise Woman, an Internationally recognised and respected authority in adrenal burnout and preventative health. She has been a naturopath, speaker and trainer for more than 3 decades and is the "Sovereign of Simplifying" complex health topics Jen gives you the BAM, the Bare Arse Minimum, making it easy to integrate sustainable change to your life. She wants people to understand the basics as they are our foundation and when the foundation is solid, we flourish.

Experiencing corporate burnout in her 20's, eventually a car accident stopped her in her tracks, and she knew she could not go back to the way she had been living and working. It was through natural therapies that she was able to rise out of adrenal burnout. Jennifer was so inspired; she went back to school to study to be a naturopath specialising into how "day to day" life stressors impact our physical, emotional and mental health.

Having experienced corporate burnout firsthand, Jennifer now works closely with some of the world's most well-known brands to restore work life balance and minimise presenteeism and absenteeism in their organisations.

Subscribing to the philosophy that wealth and success mean nothing without your health, Jennifer authored F*CK The Stress and fourteen other health-related titles, sharing practical real-life strategies to help teams and individuals improve their health, wellbeing and productivity by finding balance in their lives. Jennifer is also the host of Healthy Life Hacks Podcast and co-host of Smart Sassy Seniors Podcast with her wife Alice.

At 63, Jennifer is the realistic health practitioner and speaker for today's workplace and world.

She is known for her fun, humorous, no-nonsense approach to healthy living, and her proven ability to motivate others to make positive changes to their lives both inside and outside the workplace, Jennifer is a highly sought after presenter, speaking to corporations globally for more than twenty years.

Self-described as a psychedelic, peace and brown rice loving hippie and a passionate, adventurous traveler, when Jennifer isn't writing or speaking, you will find her surfing or gardening and focused to help leave the world a better place.

Determined to leave the world a better place, Jennifer has also established The Q Foundation to give health, hope and happiness to children in poverty-stricken countries through providing education, health care, accommodation and welfare services.

www.ingramcontent.com/pod-product-compliance
Lightning Source LLC
Chambersburg PA
CBHW042049290426
44110CB00001B/6